CHICAGO PUBLIC LIBRARY
BUSINESS / SCIENCE / TECHNOLOGY
400 S. STATE ST.   60605

D1110258

Rehabilitation
and Continuity of Care
in Pulmonary Disease

BUSINESS / SCIENCE / TECHNOLOGY DIVISION
CHICAGO PUBLIC LIBRARY
400 SOUTH STATE STREET
CHICAGO, IL 60605

Rehabilitation and Continuity of Care in Pulmonary Disease

DONALD F. MAY

Assistant Professor
Department of Cardiopulmonary Care Sciences
Georgia State University

Faculty Lecture Series in Respiratory Care

JOHN W. YOUTSEY, Editor

Associate Dean
School of Allied Health Professions
Georgia State University

with 79 illustrations

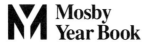 **Mosby Year Book**

St. Louis   Baltimore   Boston   Chicago   London   Philadelphia   Sydney   Toronto

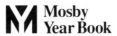

Mosby
Year Book

Dedicated to Publishing Excellence

Editor: David Marshall
Assistant Editor: Christy Mangold
Project Manager: Mark Spann
Production Editor: Christine M. Ripperda
Productionist: Kathy Teal
Book Design: Candace Conner
Cover Design: David Zielinski

Copyright © 1991 by Mosby–Year Book, Inc.
A Mosby imprint of Mosby–Year Book, Inc.

All rights reserved. No part of this publication may be reproduced,
stored in a retrieval system, or transmitted, in any form or by any
means, electronic, mechanical, photocopying, recording, or otherwise,
without prior written permission from the publisher.

Printed in the United States of America

Mosby–Year Book, Inc.
11830 Westline Industrial Drive
St. Louis, Missouri 63146

Library of Congress Cataloging-in-Publication Data

May, Donald F.
    Rehabilitation and continuity of care in pulmonary disease / Donald F. May.
        p.   cm. — (Faculty lecture series in respiratory care)
    Includes bibliographical references and index.
    ISBN 0-8016-5679-6
    1.   Respiratory organs—Diseases—Patients—Long term care.
2.   Respiratory organs—Diseases—Patients—Rehabilitation.
I.   Title.   II.   Series.
    [DNLM: 1.   Chronic Disease—rehabilitation.   2.   Home Care Services.
3.   Long Term Care.   4.   Lung Diseases—rehabilitation.   WF 600
M466r]
RC732.M39   1991
616.2'406—dc20
DNLM/DLC
for Library of Congress   90-13324
                                                                                   CIP

VT/MV   9   8   7   6   5   4   3

CHICAGO PUBLIC LIBRARY
BUSINESS / SCIENCE / TECHNOLOGY
400 S. STATE ST.   60605

R0l1qq 42b34

To my wife and best friend,
Ruth Ann May, and to my children,
Daniel, Rebekah, Sarah, and Deborah

Preface _____

This text is written for those beginning the study of long-term care and rehabilitation of patients with a chronic pulmonary disorder. It began as a series of lectures to different groups of health-care practitioners involved in rehabilitation. Respiratory therapists, physical therapists, nurses, and other health-care personnel will find useful material in this text. Those working in home care and providing durable medical equipment to patients, but not having a strong background in health care, will find many topics in the text instructive.

In 1977 I began work in pulmonary rehabilitation with a good background in acute respiratory care and little knowledge of rehabilitation, aside from patient education. For 6 months before beginning an outpatient rehabilitation program I immersed myself in the literature and communicated with as many people as I could identify working in the area. From this study, and subsequent experience, I came to appreciate the complex nature of rehabilitation, the important role of the patient in the process, and the necessity of a team approach to long-term care.

Much of what I now know about rehabilitation and home care I learned as I went through the process with each patient. The patient, the patient's family, the physician, and the health-care practitioners involved in the program all learned together. We quickly found that none of us had all the answers and that by working in concert the patient received the greatest benefit from our corporate knowledge and care. The patient and the patient's family became the focus of our team efforts, and together we all struggled toward the goal of optimizing the functional capacity of the one suffering from the pulmonary disorder.

I extend my appreciation to the hundreds of patients with whom I have had a professional and personal relationship and to the students who over the years have cared enough to be challenged, to grow, and in turn to teach as well as learn. Thank you for being a part of this work.

Donald F. May

Acknowledgments ————————————

The author wishes to acknowledge the following individuals and corporations for their assistance, input, guidance, and influence in the writing of this text.

- The hundreds of patients with whom I have had a professional and personal relationship.
- The students who have cared enough to be challenged, to grow, and in turn to teach as well as learn.
- My colleagues and friends:

Ms. Roberta Dismukes, R.N.
Ms. Nancy Smith, R.R.T.
Ms. Carol Mercer, R.N.
Mr. Christopher Kennedy, R.R.T.
Mr. Lee Wilhelm, R.R.T.
Ms. Laura Blackwell, R.N.
Mr. Joseph Harrelson, R.R.T.
Ms. Lisa McLeash
Mr. Paul Brown
Raymond Dillon, D.B.A.
David Martin, Ph.D.
John Youtsey, Ph.D., R.R.T.
Michael Belman, M.D.
Bruce Cassidy, M.D.
William Kenney, M.D.

- Piedmont Hospital, Atlanta, Georgia
Glasrock Home Health Care of Atlanta
Travenol Respiratory Home Care of Atlanta

Contents _____

SECTION II

SECTION III

6

Medication and diet in treatment of pulmonary disorders, 95

7

Mechanical ventilation, oxygen equipment, and care of equipment in the home, 114

8

Performing respiratory care in the home, 136

9

Discharge planning and community resources in pulmonary rehabilitation, 155

10

The home-care company and durable medical equipment in home care, 169

Appendix

List of frequently used acronyms in *Rehabilitation and Continuity of Care in Pulmonary Disease* ————————

ABG	Arterial Blood Gas
ADL	Activities of Daily Living
AV	Audiovisual
BPM	Beats Per Minute (cardiac)
COPD	Chronic Obstructive Pulmonary Disease
CORF	Comprehensive Outpatient Rehabilitation Facility
DLCO	Diffusion Capacity for Carbon Monoxide in the Lungs
DME	Durable Medical Equipment
HR	Heart Rate
IBW	Ideal Body Weight
ICU	Intensive Care Unit
I:E	Ratio of time for Inspiration to Expiration
IPPB	Intermittent Positive Pressure Breathing
L/min	Liters per Minute
MDI	Metered-Dose Inhaler
MET	Metabolic Equivalent
MSVC	Maximum Sustained Ventilatory Capacity
MVV	Maximum Voluntary Ventilation
OTC	Over-the-Counter
psig	Pounds per Square Inch Gauge
RER	Respiratory Exchange Ratio
RQ	Respiratory Quotient
RR	Respiratory Rate
SOB	Shortness of Breath
SVC	Slow Vital Capacity
USN	Ultrasonic Nebulizer
V_E	Minute Ventilation (same as $\dot{V}_E$)
V_{O_2}	Oxygen Consumption (same as $\dot{V}_{O_2}$)
V_{CO_2}	Carbon Dioxide Production (same as $\dot{V}_{CO_2}$)
$V_{O_2\ max}$	Maximum Oxygen Consumption (same as $\dot{V}_{O_2\ max}$)
$V_{CO_2\ max}$	Maximum Carbon Dioxide Production (same as $\dot{V}_{CO_2\ max}$)
$V_{O_2\ eq}$	Ventilatory Equivalent for Oxygen (same as $\dot{V}_{O_2\ eq}$)
$V_{CO_2\ eq}$	Ventilatory Equivalent for Carbon Dioxide (same as $\dot{V}_{CO_2\ eq}$)
VRE	Ventilation Retraining Exercise
WOB	Work of Breathing

CHAPTER **1**

Introduction and overview

PREVALENCE OF CHRONIC RESPIRATORY CONDITIONS

The incidence of respiratory disorders in the United States has been increasing over the past several decades (Table 1-1). Although atmospheric pollution is prevalent, its role in causing respiratory disease is yet unclear. But cigarette smoking is recognized as one of the greatest contributing factors in the development of respiratory disorders and heart disease. Though the percentage of people in the United States who smoke is smaller than it was 20 years ago, millions of people continue to smoke. It has been estimated that approximately 1 million people take up smoking each year. In 1983 more than 600 billion cigarettes were consumed in the United States. In the 1960s more than 50% of adult males and more than 33% of adult females smoked cigarettes. Today the smoking habit is about equally distributed among males and females. In 1985 it was reported that there were more teenage females smoking than teenage males and that deaths of women from lung cancer now exceed deaths from breast cancer. We are only beginning to appreciate the harmful effects of secondhand smoke on nonsmokers. It may take 20 to 30 years for a respiratory disease associated with cigarette smoking to develop; therefore, respiratory disorders will continue to be a major health problem in society well into the next century.

DISEASE VS. DISABILITY

Health-care services most often direct patient-care efforts toward relief of the patient's immediate complaint. Too often little effort is directed at reducing disabilities caused by the disease. Health care should be directed at reducing symptoms *and* disabilities. Acute care generally focuses on the symptoms of the disorder with the ultimate goal being a "cure." On the other hand, rehabilitation emphasizes lifestyle

1

Table 1-1 Prevalence of major chronic respiratory conditions among the civilian population in the United States*†

Condition	Bronchitis	Emphysema	Asthma	Bronchitis	Emphysema	Asthma
		1970			1979-1983	
% Seeing physician	93.8	97.0	95.8	94.9	96.3	96.7
% Limited in activity	4.0	44.9	17.1	4.7	48.2	21.3
					1985	
Persons reporting	6,526	1,313	6,031	11,974	1,993	11,621
Male	2,999	990	3,047	4,326	1,448	3,064
Female	3,527	323	2,984	7,292	627	4,784
White	6,031	1,290	5,167	10,428	1,942	7,425
Other	495	‡	864	1,093	115	1,119
					1989	
Number per 1,000 of total U.S. population	32.7	6.6	30.2	49.2	8.2	47.7
<18 years	2,592	‡	2,075	3,235	‡	3,901
18-44 years	1,691	136	1,906	4,641	123	4,302
45-64 years	1,462	575	1,369	2,476	795	1,914
>65 years	782	602	681	1,622	1,062	1,504

*Data obtained from the National Health Interview Survey, National Center for Health Statistics, U.S. Department of Health and Human Services.
†All data reported in thousands, except number per 1,000 of total U.S. population.
‡Data do not meet standards of reliability or precision.

changes that will enable the patient to maximize his potential. Respiratory-care practitioners can play a major role in all aspects of care for the patient with a chronic pulmonary disorder.

To assess our own attitudes toward the care we provide, we can ask ourselves: Should care and therapy be directed at the pathophysiologic changes in the organ system affected by the disease, or should they be directed at the physical manifestations of the pulmonary disorder? The answer to this question will be different for the various health-care disciplines. It will also depend on the state of the disorder at the time. In acute care the disease process and symptoms become the primary focus of medical care; the disabilities and the lifestyle changes resulting from the disorder are not the first priority in the treatment plan. Historically our medical system has been designed to care for patients suffering from acute illnesses. The result is that fewer resources have been allocated for chronic care.

An initial assessment of the patient's condition is necessary to create the foundation for care and rehabilitation. An accurate diagnosis and establishment of baseline physical measurements are essential for a successful program. It is important to include an assessment of physical findings and the behavior of the patient and his family, for example, how the patient and his family have adjusted to the patient's condition. The patient's adaptation to his symptoms will affect how well the care program will be carried out. Acute problems, such as bronchospasm, excessive secretions, and inflammation, often can be controlled effectively through medication and therapy. In a comprehensive rehabilitation program, it is ultimately the patient who assumes responsibility for his own compliance and success. Patients with chronic disorders can be expected to return to the physician's office or appear in the emergency room with recurring acute problems. The patient and family should understand that effective long-term care also requires the rapid recognition and resolution of acute problems.

Many factors contribute to the focus of the health-care system on the symptoms of a disease rather than on the disabilities and lifestyle changes it causes. The American health-care system traditionally has had a strong foundation in acute care rather than in long-term or chronic care. Labeled by his disease, a patient with a chronic disorder often loses his identity as a person. Unfortunately the number of people requiring care often limits the time a health-care professional, especially in an acute-care facility, can spend getting familiar with each patient. The high degree of specialization in medicine may also contribute to a focus on a specific symptom of a disease rather than on the broad effects of the disease on behavior. It is important that all members of the health-care team understand that the patient and family often tend to concentrate on the symptoms that are most uncomfortable. Once these primary symptoms are relieved, other aspects of the health-care plan, such as maintenance care, nutrition, and exercise, are often forgotten.

After a care plan has been developed to relieve or minimize physical symptoms, attention must be given to the psychologic, emotional, and physical disabilities associated with the medical problem. Home care should be considered an extension of hospital care. In the hospital the patient is dependent on the medical staff for correct, timely, and thorough application of a prescribed medical program. At home the patient will be assigned the same tasks, though he had not had such responsibilities while in the hospital. This change in role can contribute to poor compliance with the health-care plan. The patient is often asked to take home a complicated array of pills, other medications, and treatments. These therapies must be incorporated along with therapeutic exercises and perhaps dietary changes into a relatively disciplined pattern of living. In addition to creating a disruption in the patient's lifestyle, the home-care program may be difficult for the patient to comply with because of his disabilities. Support services, such as follow-up phone calls or a reassessment of the medical program within 24 to 48 hours after discharge, are necessary. The chronic nature of a pulmonary disease requires that medical care be provided with consideration for the patient's lifestyle and warrants the early introduction of rehabilitation activities into the acute-care setting.

PROGRAM STRUCTURES FOR PULMONARY REHABILITATION

In 1981 the executive committee of the American Thoracic Society (ATS) and the medical section of the American Lung Association (ALA) adopted a statement on pulmonary rehabilitation (Appendix I). This statement defined pulmonary rehabilitation, addressed the sequence of rehabilitation activities, identified both the essential and additional services that might be included in a pulmonary rehabilitation program, and presented the benefits and limitations of rehabilitation in a pulmonary disorder.

Rehabilitation activities can be incorporated into three different aspects of the health-care system: in-patient care, out-patient care, and home care. In each setting the approach taken will have advantages and disadvantages. As is true in most areas of medicine, there is no single way in which a patient can or should be rehabilitated. Rehabilitation is an art as well as a science. The decision on which or how many approaches to utilize for a given patient will depend on the resources available, the physical condition of the patient, and the willingness and ability of the patient and family to cooperate. The lack of physical facilities in a health-care institution should not be a major limitation when considering the implementation of a pulmonary rehabilitation program. The commitment of the health-care professionals is the most important element in developing a pulmonary rehabilitation program.

The structure of the rehabilitation program should be one that accommodates the needs and lifestyle of the patient and family. The patient may be less concerned about specific program activities than he is about how he will be able to carry on daily activities, such as shopping for food or cleaning the house. The patient's ability to perform such tasks will have a major influence on the success of any rehabilitation program and should be considered during the planning process. Before a rehabilitation program is implemented, the patient, the family, and the health-care team must discuss all facets of the program.

The plan for rehabilitation should address the following areas: goals of the patient and family, emotional status of the patient and family, financial aspects of long-term care, support networks and social outlets that may or may not exist, misunderstandings and the need for information, job-related problems, long-term prognosis, and the necessity and planning of follow-up care.

Through education and training, which eliminate ignorance and provide skills for self-care, rehabilitation can effect change in a patient's behavior. But it takes a great deal of effort and time—much more time than, for instance, an 8-day hospitalization—to bring about a change in well-established behavior. When the patient or family is available only for a short period of time, the emphasis should be on education and training in self-care skills. For this reason the emphasis of in-patient rehabilitation activities should be on educating and training the patient and family.

In-patient care and rehabilitation

In-patient care and rehabilitation is most often initiated after the patient is admitted to the hospital for treatment of an acute exacerbation. Rehabilitation activities should begin in earnest once the patient's medical condition has stabilized. However, in most instances the rehabilitation process can begin upon admission. Education and training are the primary activities of the in-patient rehabilitation program, and they can be done with the family even if the patient cannot participate. Goals should be centered around immediate needs and short-term results. Every effort should be made to allow the patient and family to perform the prescribed therapy and to be responsible, with guidance, for administration of prescribed medication. The greatest difference between in-patient and other rehabilitation programs is the number and types of goals established.

In some in-patient rehabilitation programs, patients are admitted directly into the program while they are relatively symptom-free. The patient stays in the hospital for 10 days to 2 weeks, learning and practicing various program activities, thus preparing for self-care at home. Hospitalization provides an excellent opportunity for education and training under controlled conditions. The family should be involved as much as possible in administering treatments, deciding about care, and sharing information. The goals established for the patient should be clear, measurable, and short term, and the patient should have major input in goal development. Such patient involvement encourages "ownership" of the responsibility for treatment and increases the likelihood of compliance with a rehabilitation program. Care must be taken to personalize the training in program activities and emphasize the application of these activities in the patient's home. Follow-up after discharge, consisting of a phone call or a letter, is a very important method of reinforcement of the established care plan.

Out-patient care and rehabilitation

A second approach to meeting the needs of the patient is an out-patient program. This program structure is often administered through a hospital's out-patient ambulatory services, emergency department, or clinic. It may even be an extension of the department of respiratory care, where pulmonary rehabilitation or respiratory care treatments are generally provided as one of many clinic services. With an emphasis on long-term care, a planned out-patient program can be comprehensive and quite involved. Out-patient rehabilitation programs often cover a broad scope of activities and rehabilitation modalities, many of which are not included as part of in-patient programs. Because of the greater amount of time the patient spends in an out-patient program, it should be more comprehensive and intensive. Goals should emphasize changes in behavior and lifestyle. Progress is generally evident to the staff and the patient throughout the course of the program. Follow-up visits to the clinic or the physician's office are a routine, accepted part of the program. Frequent visits promote cooperation among all members of the health-care team—patient, physician, and rehabilitation staff. The box on p. 6 gives examples of schedules that may be used in an out-patient rehabilitation program.

Using the sample schedule in the box on p. 6, a number of patients can be scheduled to participate in the program on alternating days: Monday, Wednesday, and

SAMPLE SCHEDULE OF
REHABILITATION MODALITIES IN AN OUT-PATIENT PROGRAM

The patient is to take all morning medications and treatments before coming to the rehabilitation program for the session. He should spend 3½ to 4 hours in the facility. More time may be required to allow for rests or additonal therapies or exercises.

Morning patient

9:00 AM Arrive. Rest while staff reviews daily diary, activity sheet and medication schedule, etc.
Counsel patient (Alter schedule as needed.) on aspects of self-care and activities as observed from review of material and comments. (Family attends.)

9:30 AM Education/training session; therapy and various informational items are discussed. (Family attends.)

10:00 AM Exercise training/therapy session; strength and/or endurance activities: calisthenics, resistive work, treadmill, bicycle, stairs, walking.

11:00 AM Ventilation retraining exercises: modified calisthenics, diaphragmatic breathing, pursed-lip breathing, control of breathing with activities of daily living.

11:30 AM Respiratory therapy TX, bronchial hygiene, etc.

12:00 PM Various individual needs: occupational therapy, nutritional needs, pharmacy or physician visit, self-care, care of equipment, work efficiency, schedule planning, review of program activities and home activities.

12:30 PM Exit. Do lab work (if needed).

•   •   •

Afternoon patient

1:00 PM Arrive. Rest while staff reviews daily diary, etc.
Other activities and intervals repeat as outlined above.

4:30 PM Exit. Do lab work (if needed).

Friday one week and Tuesday, Thursday, and Saturday the next week. On nonprogram days the patient should perform all activities at home but spread them out over the day as he will be expected to perform them after the program has been completed. This routine for scheduled visits to the rehabilitation program is continued throughout the 6 to 8 weeks of the formal program.

At times it will be beneficial to the patient to be "weaned" from the formal program. For example, if the patient is not confident of his ability or has little support at home for self-care, the above schedule can be tapered to fewer visits per week over an extended period of time, for example, Tuesday and Thursday visits for 2 weeks, then one visit a week for 2 weeks, then one visit every 30 days. Follow-up can be done as needed, but some contact should be made at least every 2 or 3 months. This contact can be made by telephone or letter, but in some cases a visit to the home may be best. Once the staff gets to know the patient, the follow-up method can be determined. The objective of a follow-up program is to maintain open channels of communication and to encourage the patient and assess his condition and compliance with the care plan. The patient's visit to the physician's office is another opportunity for follow-up. The care plan and all reports, schedules, and test results are forwarded to the referring (primary) physician, who is ultimately responsible for long-term care and follow-up.

Home care and rehabilitation

A third approach to rehabilitation is *home care*. This type of program is frequently a result of participation in either the in-patient or out-patient program. Home-care programs are very individualized and long range and are less intense than either of the other types of program structures. The patient and family assume the responsibility for carrying out the activities in the program, monitoring themselves and recording the results. Often the only resource available to the patient during home care is the physician's office. If progress is to continue, the patient must take charge of his own rehabilitation with minimal encouragement and coaching. Unfortunately, when the patient visits his physician, the emphasis is often on providing immediate care rather than rehabilitation assistance.

Companies that supply medical equipment for use in the home can be an asset to home care by having their professional staff visit the patient's home to reinforce activities and monitor progress. If the home-care program is begun after the out-patient rehabilitation program, the out-patient program should communicate the rehabilitation program's goals and therapies to the home-care company. The home-care company can be valuable to the patient by bringing into the home rehabilitation services and personnel usually found only at a health-care facility. The staff of the home-care company is able to reinforce skills already learned and provide practical suggestions for the application of techniques. The company can help with follow-up and make suggestions to the physician for program alterations, thus improving communication and the likelihood of patient compliance.

Rehabilitation is dynamic, so health-care professionals should feel free to be creative when designing programs for individual patients. A rehabilitation program should not necessarily have a particular format. A "cookbook" approach to individual problems should be avoided in rehabilitation. Whatever structure is used in a rehabilitation program, it should provide a framework for addressing the individual's needs in an efficient manner. It must involve the patient in decision-making and foster in the patient a sense of personal responsibility for his own health care.

INDIVIDUALIZATION OF PATIENT EDUCATION AND REHABILITATION

Pulmonary rehabilitation programs should contain essential elements from each area of what can be called the "wheel of rehabilitation" (Fig. 1-1). Rehabilitation techniques and the sequence and timing of activities must be tailored to the specific

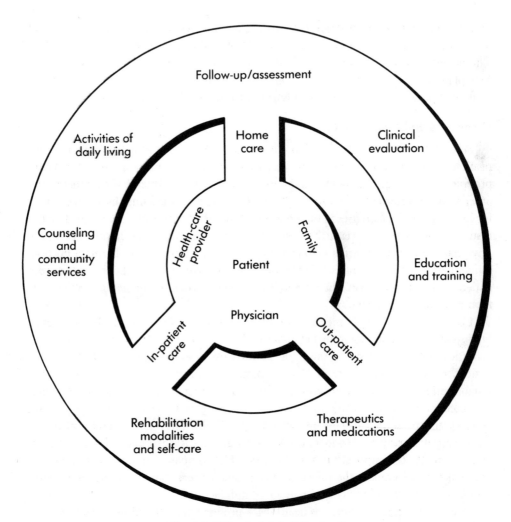

Fig. 1-1 "Wheel of Rehabilitation."

needs and desires of the patient. The objective is to return the individual to the highest functional capacity possible, increase self-esteem, and optimize the patient's medical care. The patient must play an integral part in program activities and be committed to following through with the rehabilitation plan. The patient is the *key member* of the health-care team involved with his rehabilitation.

It is important to remember that the atmosphere of a hospital or other health-care facility is foreign to most people and that a transition must be made between "real" life at home and life in the hospital. The patient must take what he has learned in the hospital and implement it where he lives and works. Home visits by members of the rehabilitation staff and other methods of follow-up can be important in promoting

---

THE ACCP-ATS DEFINITION OF PULMONARY REHABILITATION

The art of medical practice wherein an individually tailored, multidisciplinary program is formulated which through accurate diagnosis, therapy, emotional support and education stabilizes or reverses both the physio- and psycho-pathology of pulmonary diseases and attempts to return the patient to the highest possible functional capacity allowed by his pulmonary handicap and overall life situation.

---

patient compliance. *The key element in the long-term success of a program of rehabilitation and self-care is the patient's confidence in his own ability to administer such care.*

The American College of Chest Physicians (ACCP) and the ATS have developed a working definition of pulmonary rehabilitation (see box above).

As an art pulmonary rehabilitation is open to interpretation, modification, and creativity in its application. Each program must be tailored to the needs of the individual so that each patient becomes a study in himself. Basic principles and procedures may be applied to the majority of patients, but individual needs must be the focus. As the wheel in Fig. 1-1 illustrates, the patient can have access to any of the resources in rehabilitation according to his needs.

Pulmonary rehabilitation is process-oriented rather than product-oriented. There is no set sequence to follow in the rehabilitation process. The most basic and important step in any pulmonary rehabilitation program—and the one on which all others depend—is the determination of an accurate diagnosis. The therapeutics, procedures, support networks, and educational goals require that the health team know what it is facing. It is important to know the specific disorder a patient has and the extent to which it has progressed. Defining the patient's medical status will allow the staff to recognize signs to monitor for change and will assist the staff in determining a prognosis. It is also possible with this information to make program objectives clear, realistic, and relevant. The intent of rehabilitative care is to minimize further deterioration of the patient's condition, relieve symptoms, and maximize the patient's functional capacity. Ultimately the patient should be able to care for himself and to function at the level he desires within the limits of his disorder. The patient should have significant input into the development of program goals. More importantly, he must decide the quality of his own life. The patient with a pulmonary disorder should understand that he will find himself somewhere within the wheel of rehabilitation as long as he is receiving health care.

CONTINUITY OF CARE AND REHABILITATION

On the rim of the wheel of rehabilitation (Fig. 1-1) are the many aspects of rehabilitation as they pertain to the patient with a pulmonary disorder. The spokes of the wheel are the three rehabilitation structures in which a patient may find himself during the years he is dealing with his disorder: in-patient care, out-patient care, and home care. With any one of these program formats, a patient can receive the various services that are part of pulmonary rehabilitation. A patient with a pulmonary disorder will always find himself somewhere within this wheel if he is receiving health care. A primary objective of rehabilitation is that the patient, once trained and competent in self-care, will use only necessary health-care services as designated by his physician.

At the center of the wheel is the patient with a pulmonary disorder, his family, the physician, and other health-care providers supporting the patient and his family. The patient is the focus of rehabilitation efforts and is involved in making decisions about his program of care, for example, accessing resources and choosing which parts of the rehabilitation program to implement and when to implement them. The relationship between patient and physician is crucial to the success of rehabilitation. A physician's positive and supportive attitude increases the likelihood that the patient will comply with the prescribed program and maximize his own recovery.

A thorough evaluation is essential before any rehabilitation program can begin. Data from this evaluation helps the physician make a firm diagnosis and establishes a baseline from which to monitor progress. Many areas can be assessed, but it is important that a good clinical evaluation and psychologic assessment be made. Particular attention should be paid to the patient's lifestyle, living conditions, and daily habits, as well as his coping behaviors and the possible existence of depression. The clinical evaluation should include a physical examination, diagnostic tests, personal history, occupational history, and family history. Complete diagnostic testing should include full pulmonary function tests, chest films, a cardiac assessment, and clinical laboratory tests.

Another important aspect of a rehabilitation program is the medication prescribed by the physician. Poor compliance with a prescribed medication regimen often contributes to the worsening of a patient's condition. A written schedule of all medications, such as a check-off sheet, can serve as a reminder to the patient. This schedule should be considered part of the prescription process. To optimize each dosage and minimize the side effects of medications, the health-care team should be assured that the prescription is being followed as written. When this schedule is incorporated into the patient's daily diary, a good assessment of the effect of medications and treatments on the patient's lifestyle and symptoms is possible. Because of the many medications and treatments used to relieve symptoms of a pulmonary disorder, it is often difficult for the patient to keep medications organized without a written schedule.

An educational strategy should be developed to train the patient and his family to administer medications and perform various rehabilitation and self-care tasks. Without proper, consistent instruction, it will be difficult to attain short- or long-term goals and to reap all of the potential benefits of the patient's care plan. Sharing information is only one part of the education process, and education is only one part of rehabilitation. The patient must be able to make the information he receives practical and apply it in a personal way. This implementation can be enhanced by an involved health-care staff and open discussions among the patient, his family, and the staff. These discussions can take place in classroom sessions, in group meetings with other patients, and in one-on-one sessions that help the patient develop various psychomotor skills. An educational setting can provide a means of recognizing and rewarding desired behavior. Such encouragement promotes development in the patient and his family of a positive attitude toward healthful living.

To achieve desired goals, pulmonary rehabilitation involves a variety of therapies, treatments, and activities. For example, training in control and coordination of breathing can be beneficial to participation in the activities of daily living. The training and therapeutic modalities used in rehabilitation may be applicable in treating only certain disorders. For example, pursed-lip breathing may be helpful to the very elderly and can be beneficial to patients with obstructive disorders, but it is not useful in treating patients with purely restrictive disorders. It is the responsibility of the director of the rehabilitation program, along with the physician, to ensure that the patient is receiving the appropriate components of his care plan. The modalities most frequently included in a rehabilitation program are ventilation retraining, reconditioning exercises, bronchial hygiene techniques, relaxation therapy, equipment care and operation, and self-care efficiency principles. Other aspects of care may be required to assist the patient, such as marital counseling or financial assistance.

Counseling of patient and family is a vital part of long-term care and rehabilitation. Most health-care practitioners are not professional counselors, so when psychologic or emotional problems are evident, they should seek assistance from a qualified professional. However, a hospital's rehabilitation staff often know the patient on a more intimate level than other hospital staff and, as a result, often find themselves in a counseling role. The most important skill in counseling is the ability to listen. Acquiring this skill may require rehabilitation staff to be trained as sensitive, intelligent listeners. A great deal of the information obtained by the staff from the patient can be shared with a counseling professional. However, even if information is not transmitted to a professional counselor, the act of listening demonstrates concern and sincerity on the part of the staff.

Patient and family counseling done by the rehabilitation staff usually involves recognizing a problem and matching it to the necessary community resource. Medical social workers are an important asset in identifying resources for the patient, but the patient needs to learn to identify and access resources for himself. Counseling can also involve making suggestions to improve compliance with program activities and alterations in lifestyle. Many of the patient's problems and the family's concerns may be brought up while discussing a rehabilitation activity, such as an aspect of the medication schedule, or the daily diaries used in the program. Reviewing schedules and diaries can provide an opportunity for an open discussion of how the patient feels about the program, his disabilities, or his family.

The philosophy of the rehabilitation staff should be to "work themselves out of a job." Most of the health-care services provided for the patient, such as respiratory treatments, exercises, and equipment operation, must be learned and eventually performed by the patient alone. Performing the self-care involved in rehabilitation may be the first of several steps by the patient toward his full participation as a member of the health-care team. The patient should participate in the adaptation of activities, treatments, and exercises to his own lifestyle and living environment. Such participation is a major step in rehabilitation and requires much effort and frequent follow-up, modification, and reinforcement. By encouraging a personalized program of activities and maintaining open communication, the health-care staff can help the patient incorporate rehabilitation activities into his lifestyle.

Follow-up of the patient involved in pulmonary self-care is essential if long-term benefits are to be derived. As illustrated in Fig. 1-1, the patient with a chronic pulmonary disorder will always find himself at some point in the wheel throughout his lifetime. More activity and greater commitment will be needed at some points than at others, but at no time should access to assistance not be available. The decision about what methods of rehabilitation are needed is made by the patient and his family together with the physician during follow-up. It is often during a visit to the physician's office, the most common form of follow-up, that problems or the need for retraining are identified. Follow-up also provides a good opportunity for the physician to reinforce behaviors and to encourage the patient in his performance of self-care.

BENEFITS OF PULMONARY REHABILITATION

For years papers have been published describing rehabilitation programs for patients with pulmonary disorders and the programs' varying degrees of success. These programs have provided documentation of the benefits to be realized by patients involved in pulmonary rehabilitation. Although objective improvements in the parameters of pulmonary function are not frequently found, many patients have reported fewer symptomatic complaints. Patients are able to function at a higher level in their daily activities and have demonstrated increased tolerance of stress and reduction in acute exacerbations resulting in hospitalization. The inability of rehabilitation to repair damaged lung tissue and halt the deterioration of pulmonary function caused by the disease should not be viewed as failure of the rehabilitation process. The goal of rehabilitation is not to cure the pulmonary disorder but to restore the patient's lifestyle and physical condition to an optimum level within the limits of the disorder. Some of the documented benefits of pulmonary rehabilitation are given in the box on p. 13.

A patient with a pulmonary disorder who is participating in a rehabilitation program will continue to have the disease and experience exacerbations that manifest the characteristics of the disease. This situation is similar to that of a patient with paralysis, who functions at a higher level and experiences fewer problems after rehabilitation.

_____ BENEFITS OF PULMONARY REHABILITATION _____

- Decrease in frequency and duration of hospitalizations
- Socioeconomic advantages, such as a return to the work force
- Reduction in anxiety levels and depression
- Reduction in somatic concerns
- Improved ability to contribute to family and society
- Improved self-esteem
- Slower rate of deterioration in pulmonary function
- Improved exercise tolerance
- Increased survival and longevity

MOTIVATING THE PATIENT WITH A PULMONARY DISORDER

Once the patient's problem has been diagnosed and a program of activities and its goals have been set, how does the health-care team keep the patient motivated to continue the rehabilitation program? Both patient and staff can put forth a great deal of effort during an 8-week in-patient program, but their efforts will be futile if the patient discontinues program activities once at home. Several strategies can be employed to keep the patient motivated: beginning the program slowly, setting reasonable goals, documenting the patient's efforts, and showing enthusiasm. Because nothing breeds success like success, the patient will be motivated to work at the rehabilitation process as he observes improvement.

Different strategies for motivation can be extremely important when symptoms vary with the change of seasons or when a change in the patient's daily routine causes a lapse in scheduled rehabilitation activities. The box on p. 14 lists strategies that have been helpful in motivating people with pulmonary disorders to continue a supervised rehabilitation program or to continue unsupervised rehabilitation and self-care activities at home.

A daily diary kept by the patient is an important tool for documenting the rehabilitation process. If a patient is not used to keeping a log of activities, the daily diary should be simple and straightforward. Some training and practice in using the diary will be required, and a discussion of the diary at each visit with the hospital's rehabilitation staff will be necessary. The patient should record on two or three lines what he did at each point, for example, every 2 hours, throughout the day. By doing so, the patient will produce a useful diary and build an appreciation for the usefulness of it. This information can be helpful when identifying potential times for rehabilitation activities at home or when scheduling medications and meals. A diary of symptoms kept over several weeks can characterize the pulmonary disorder for the patient in terms of coughing, sputum production, episodes of shortness of breath, etc. Several weeks of a diary will provide a means for assessing changes in the patient's condition

```
┌─────────────────────────────────────────────────────────────────────────┐
│ ──── IMPROVING COMPLIANCE WITH REHABILITATION ACTIVITIES ────             │
│                                                                           │
│   Patient should:                                                         │
│   • Maintain a daily diary                                                │
│   • Openly discuss reasons for not following the program                  │
│   • Participate in establishing program goals                             │
│   • Establish a goal-attainment record                                    │
│   • Adhere to agreed-upon objectives                                      │
│                                                                           │
│   Program staff should:                                                   │
│   • Make the benefits of rehabilitation clearly understood                │
│   • Describe in detail the activities in the program                      │
│   • Revise the program if the patient voices strong resistance            │
│   • Answer all questions                                                  │
│   • Be organized and professional                                         │
│   • Provide for follow-up care, such as home visits                       │
│   • Involve the patient's physician in the program                        │
└─────────────────────────────────────────────────────────────────────────┘
```

and making adjustments to program activities. The patient should be given one page for each day and encouraged to record any and all observations and feelings he desires. During each of the patient's visits to the hospital, program staff should spend 15 minutes going over the diary and other forms completed by the patient. The diary and forms should be discussed, and observations should be made by the staff, identifying areas of need and making appropriate suggestions.

The patient in rehabilitation must understand the reasons for the various activities and procedures in a program. A clear understanding of what is to be accomplished will aid in patient motivation and compliance. Short-term objectives and benefits should be clearly separated from potential long-term benefits. In this way it is possible to keep an appropriate focus on the immediate needs of the patient, such as relief of symptoms. As short-term goals are realized, a foundation of trust between the patient and the rehabilitation staff is established for future activities. By carefully establishing goals, the staff and the patient can agree on and observe some visible measure of progress. The patient can look back frequently during the program and see how far he has come and will realize the value of his efforts.

The staff of the rehabilitation program must be willing to allow the patient to control many program activities and, to some extent, the pace of the program. This control should allow the patient to refuse one activity and select from among several equally good alternatives. In this way the patient can appreciate his responsibility for the program, thereby increasing the likelihood of his compliance.

The transition from performing activities in the hospital program under staff supervision to performing them at home can be a difficult one. The patient will not realize many obstacles until he is in the home. A patient may not truly know whether he has mastered an exercise or a treatment until he does it at home on his own. A visit to the home can assist the staff of the rehabilitation program in assessing the conditions under which the patient is to perform self-care and then allowing for appropriate modifications. Because the patient is in the process of rehabilitation as long as he is under medical care (remember the "wheel") the staff of a program can become a resource to the patient and family instead of only the providers of a health-care service.

Rehabilitation and continuity of care for the patient with a pulmonary disorder is an ongoing process. The rehabilitation process includes the application of therapeutic modalities, such as aerosol treatments or postural drainage, and various activities, such as exercise and breathing retraining, appropriate to the disabilities of the patient. This individualization allows the patient, family, and physician and other health-care providers to deal with the whole person and not just to focus on a specific physical manifestation common to pulmonary disorders.

As evidenced by the material in Table 1-1, people who suffer from a pulmonary disorder are a significant part of society. Health-care professionals can help these patients to function at an optimum level within society. All of us benefit when each of the members of our society participates in and contributes to society to his full potential.

COMPREHENSIVE OUT-PATIENT REHABILITATION FACILITY

In an attempt to encourage development of out-patient rehabilitation programs that could better serve patients with long-term rehabilitation needs, the federal government enacted legislation to provide for reimbursement of services in a comprehensive out-patient rehabilitation facility (CORF). A CORF is a distinct type of health-care provider system established under Medicare, Part B. The origins of the CORF are found in the Omnibus Reconciliation Act of 1980, PL 96-499. Regulations for the implementation of this part of the act were completed and published in the Federal Register, Volume 47, No. 241, December 15, 1982, pp. 56282-56297. The interpretation and implementation of these regulations may be slightly different in each region of the country. The purpose of a CORF is to create another arm of the Medicare system, one that is broader in scope and more directed toward long-term health care than the present system. CORFs can extend the medical services outside large metropolitan centers into smaller communities.

General characteristics of a CORF

The health services of a CORF are intended for individuals who have significant potential for improvement. It is not a clinic for providing primary care to patients. The rehabilitation program established for the patient is aimed at specific goals that are achievable in a predictable period of time. Although extensions may be possible, 60 days should be sufficient time in which to achieve rehabilitation goals. The care plan for the patient must be reviewed at least every 60 days by the CORF physician. The CORF is not intended to be a long-term out-patient facility, providing care as long as the patient requires it.

Patients needing out-patient rehabilitation are referred to the facility by a physician. The referring physician must provide the CORF physician with all medical records pertinent to the patient. Both physicians also participate in the establishment of treatments and goals for the patient. Because the patient will be remanded to his care upon completion of the in-patient rehabilitation program, it is important that the referring physician be aware of the treatments the patient has received and their intended outcomes. The treatment plan is then written by the CORF physician in consultation with the CORF staff. Regular review of this plan is encouraged.

All services provided by the CORF physician or staff must be performed at the out-patient facility. The only exception is the one visit from the CORF staff to the patient's home to assess the effect of the home environment on the patient's rehabilitation goals. The CORF must be established and operated exclusively for the purpose of providing comprehensive out-patient rehabilitation services. For example, CORF cannot be an extension of an out-patient ambulatory services center. The physical plant for the CORF may be located in or with other health facilities, such as hospitals, but it must be certified and operated independently. The administrative structure and operation should be distinct from any such structures in the hospital, although the CORF may contract with a hospital for provision of some services, such as those of a clinical laboratory.

The minimum health-care services that a CORF must provide are:

Physician services

Physical-therapy services

Social or psychologic services

If the facility provides these three services, it can qualify as a CORF and apply for reimbursement through Medicare, Part B. Other health-care services that a CORF may provide and be reimbursed for are:

Occupational therapy

Speech therapy

Respiratory therapy

Nursing care

Prosthetic devices

Orthotic devices

Drugs and biologicals

Supplies, appliances, and equipment for use in the CORF

Operation of a CORF

Each patient in a comprehensive out-patient rehabilitation program needs to have the goals of his program and the services needed to achieve them delineated. Specifications for services should include the type of treatment or therapy, the frequency of application, and the anticipated duration of use. As the patient's condition changes, each aspect of the treatment plan should be evaluated and altered as necessary. The results of this review must be documented and communicated to the patient and the referring physician by the CORF staff. The CORF physician revises and reviews individual treatment plans as necessary, but at least every 60 days.

Because a CORF is a multidisciplinary health-care facility, it is important that all professional personnel coordinate their activities and that there be a free flow of information about the patient's status. Clinical records must be maintained, and particular emphasis should be paid to the status of the patient in relation to initial program goals. Regular review of patient cases should be scheduled.

The CORF building must hold all the necessary personnel, equipment, space, and supplies to implement the treatment plan designated by the CORF physician. Federal regulations governing the CORF specify minimum qualifications for personnel providing CORF services. Professionals specially trained for each service must be available at the facility at all times to ensure that all of the CORF's services are readily available. These regulations mean that the CORF cannot borrow personnel, equipment, or supplies from another facility. Each CORF must be able and prepared to carry out all plans of rehabilitation within its own facilities.

The role of health-care practitioners in a CORF

Each professional involved in patient care carries out an initial patient assessment. He also reassesses his involvement in the patient's care after any significant change in the patient's condition. Withdrawal of services is expected as the patient improves and the professional assessment indicates that the service is no longer needed.

The physician is the key ingredient in the operation of a CORF. He should be present in the facility for a sufficient amount of time to provide medical direction to the rest of the staff, establish treatment plans in rehabilitation programs, review established rehabilitation programs, participate in reviews and conferences on patient cases, and perform other medical and administrative duties.

The physical therapy offered through the CORF involves testing and measuring the function of the neuromuscular, musculoskeletal, and cardiovascular systems. Members of the physical-therapy staff are also involved in the establishment of a maintenance therapy program for the patient, as well as assessment and treatment related to dysfunctions brought about by illness or injury.

The social services offered by a CORF include the assessment of factors related to the illness and the individual's response to treatment and adjustment to care. This may include casework to resolve social or emotional problems and assessment of home situations in terms of financial resources and community resources available to the patient.

A CORF's psychologic services include assessment, diagnosis, and treatment of mental and emotional dysfunction. They also include assessment of the response of the patient to treatment and assessment of the psychologic effects of the patient's home environment.

Occupational therapy involves the teaching of techniques, evaluation of independent function, selection and teaching of therapeutic activities, and assessment of vocational rehabilitation potential. Speech therapy includes the diagnosis and treatment of speech and language disorders.

Respiratory therapy involves the assessment, treatment, and management of the health of patients with cardiopulmonary dysfunction. Therapy includes the application of techniques involved in pulmonary rehabilitation for oxygenation and ventilation. The application of therapeutic gases, aerosols, and bronchial hygiene techniques and equipment necessary for bronchial hygiene is also included in respiratory therapy, as are diagnostic tests, tests of pulmonary function and blood gases, and periodic assessments of the need for therapy. Pulmonary rehabilitation techniques such as exercise, conditioning, breathing retraining, and patient education may also be included in respiratory therapy.

Nursing services in a CORF include all nursing services specified in the treatment plan, as well as other services necessary for the achievement of rehabilitation goals.

The drugs and biologicals used in therapy must be prescribed by a physician. This is also true for some of the supplies, appliances, and equipment used in the CORF, such as nonreusable items, for example, oxygen tubes and adhesive bandages, and some durable medical equipment and appliances.

A CORF can be an excellent treatment opportunity for persons requiring outpatient rehabilitation services. In a way a CORF is a one-stop location for health-care services. Integration of all health care required by a patient can be accomplished efficiently and effectively in a CORF. This centralization of services makes help for the patient simple and accessible. The CORF is a real asset to patients in their attempt to incorporate the many and varied resources needed to deal with a complex medical problem. Follow-up is made easier, and records are centrally located for review. Furthermore, the community has an important resource for ongoing care and rehabilitation.

BIBLIOGRAPHY

Bebout DE et al: Clinical and physiological outcomes of a university-hospital pulmonary rehabilitation program, Respir Care 28(11):1468, 1983.

Bradley BL: Rehabilitation of patients with chronic respiratory disease, Respir Ther July, August 1983.

Braun SR et al: A decentralized rehabilitation program for chronic airway obstruction disease patients in small urban and rural areas of Wisconsin: a preliminary report, Public Health Rep 96(4):315-318, 1981.

Comprehensive outpatient rehabilitation facility (C.O.R.F.), Federal Register 47(241):56282-56297, 1982.

Fischer DA and Prentice WS: Feasibility of home care for certain respiratory-dependent restrictive or obstructive lung disease patients, Chest 82:739-743, 1981.

Haas A and Cardon H: Rehabilitation in chronic obstructive pulmonary disease: a 5-year study of 252 male patients, Med Clin North Am 53(3):593-606, 1969.

Hodgkin JE et al: Chronic obstructive airway diseases: current concepts in diagnosis and comprehensive care, JAMA 232(12):1243-1260, 1975.

Hodgkin JE, editor: Chronic obstructive pulmonary disease: current concepts in diagnosis and comprehensive care, 1979, American College of Chest Physicians.

Hodgkin JE, Zorn E, and Connors G: Pulmonary rehabilitation: guidelines to success, Stoneham, Mass, 1984, Butterworth Publishers.

Kane R et al: The future need for geriatric manpower in the United States, N Engl J Med 302(24):1327-1332, 1980.

Lertzman MM and Cherniack RM: Rehabilitation of patients with chronic obstructive pulmonary disease, Am Rev Respir Dis 114:1145-1165, 1976.

May DF and Kenny WR: Pulmonary rehabilitation: dealing effectively with chronic pulmonary disease, J Med Assoc Ga 69:205-208, 1980.

Miller WF: Rehabilitation of patients with chronic obstructive lung disease, Med Clin North Am 51(2):349-361, 1967.

Moser KM et al: Results of a comprehensive rehabilitation program: physiologic and functional effects on patients with chronic obstructive pulmonary disease, Arch Intern Med 140:1596-1601, 1980.

Nicol J et al: Strategies for developing a cost-effective pulmonary rehabilitation program, Respir Care 28(11):1451, 1983.

Petty TL: Pulmonary rehabilitation: better living with new techniques, Respir Care 30(2):98-107, 1985.

Petty TL and Nett LM: Pulmonary rehabilitation, Continuing Education 9(4):28-39, 1978.

Petty TL: Pulmonary rehabilitation, Basics of RD 4(1):1-6, 1975.

Petty T et al: Intensive and rehabilitative respiratory care, ed 2, Philadelphia, 1974, Lea & Febiger.

Shapiro BA et al: Rehabilitation in chronic obstructive pulmonary disease: a two-year prospective study, Respir Care 22(10):1045-1057, 1977.

Tiep B: Intensive approach to pulmonary rehabilitation, City Hope Q 8(3):6-9, 1979.

Wallace W: The road back: rehabilitating respiratory cripples, Respir Ther 43-47, March, April 1973.

Woolf CR: A rehabilitation program for improving exercise tolerance of patients with chronic lung disease, Can Med Assoc J 106:1289-1292, June 1972.

Wright RW et al: Benefits of a community–hospital rehabilitation program, Respir Care 28(11):1474, 1983.

CHAPTER 2

Developing a care plan for a
patient with a pulmonary disorder

THE PURPOSE OF A CARE PLAN

The development of a comprehensive health-care plan is not a new idea. Organizing findings from an initial assessment of a patient's condition, data from testing, results of prescribed therapeutic treatments, and notes on a patient's progress during the course of treatment is a basic part of good medical practice. However, the comprehensive approach to health care is often not followed as diligently in out-patient or rehabilitative-care settings as it would be in the acute-care setting. This lack of integration of medical information can lead to poor communication among members of a health-care team and poor coordination of patient care. Such poor communication and coordination of care ultimately can result in a program of care that is less than optimal and that is not responsive to changes in the needs of the patient and her family. It is important that a care plan be developed and communicated thoroughly to all people involved, especially to the patient.

In today's changing health-care system, coordination of services is a complex task. The complexity of self-care and the number of people seeing any one physician often diminish the physician's ability to coordinate and monitor effectively the many aspects of health care. All health-care personnel can play a role in the coordination of efforts to promote safe and effective long-term health care. As a professional a health-care worker needs to take advantage of every opportunity to assist a patient in following the care plan prescribed by her physician. Physicians need to utilize every resource at their disposal to carry out their care plan and to improve a patient's physical condition.

Comprehensive care plans are common in the acute-care setting. Problems are identified, data are gathered, desired outcomes are expressed, and therapies are instituted to relieve the patient's problem. Often this same comprehensive approach is not followed during home care. To provide continuity of care from the hospital to the home, it is essential that there be a written care plan. A primary goal in any care plan for the patient who suffers from a chronic pulmonary disorder is prevention of an acute exacerbation and subsequent rehospitalization. In today's health-care economy it is important to allocate acute-care resources wisely. If a person can perform her own care and learn to recognize problems, home care under the guidance of a physician may

---

THE PURPOSES OF A RESPIRATORY CARE PLAN

- To improve communication among the members of the health-care team
- To provide continuity of care between the hospital and the home environment
- To improve the quality of respiratory care
- To outline specific actions for the relief of acute symptoms
- To formulate long-term objectives in the treatment of the pulmonary disorder
- To establish criteria for evaluating therapies and monitoring the progression of the pulmonary disorder
- To identify education and self-care needed to allow full participation of the patient and family in the implementation of the care plan

---

eliminate a sequence of hospitalizations. The major purposes for the development of a respiratory care plan are listed in the box above.

If no care plan is written out, it will be difficult to determine whether the care prescribed for the patient has been effective and safe or needs modification. The extent to which an individual is able to participate in her own health care is a good measure of the effectiveness of the rehabilitation and the care plan. The process of education and rehabilitation should begin as soon as possible after the pulmonary disorder is identified. Too often a pulmonary disease is diagnosed in the patient's fifth decade of life. Education and rehabilitation may not be started until the disorder has become even more advanced. The early development of a respiratory care plan provides a framework for the patient and the health-care provider to know what goals to work toward, how to achieve them, and what the responsibility of each team member is to be in the future. Keeping in mind the patient's lifestyle and the characteristics of the disorder, the health-care provider can modify the plan as the patient's condition and symptoms change over time.

COMPONENTS OF THE CARE PLAN FOR PATIENTS WITH CHRONIC OBSTRUCTIVE PULMONARY DISORDER

There are many factors to consider when developing the care plan for a patient with chronic obstructive pulmonary disease (COPD). The physical and psychologic effects of the disorder must be taken into account as well as any long-term self-care activities and treatments that will be required. The plan must be individualized within the framework of the many different program structures already discussed in Chapter 1. Individualization allows the patient to feel responsible for her own care plan and solicits greater commitment from the patient to see that the objectives of the plan are carried out. Some of the more common problems to be addressed in the care plan for a COPD patient are:

ELEMENTS IN A CARE PLAN

Each of these elements can be identified for each symptom, complaint, or problem.

- The *source* of the symptom or problem, diagnosis
- Immediate *action* to be taken to relieve the symptom
- Development of *long-term goals* for care and prevention
- A method and timetable for *evaluation* of the care directed toward the symptom
- A means to *document* objective and subjective evidence for evaluation

---

Shortness of breath
Apprehension, fear, and poor coping mechanisms
Somatic concerns and poor self-concept
Inadequate nutrition and unhealthy lifestyle habits
Low tolerance of activities of daily living (ADL)
Poor compliance with parts of the care plan
    The physical aspects of the pulmonary disorder can be characterized by symptoms or problems commonly found in all patients with COPD, and each symptom or problem should be addressed in a care plan. The box above gives factors that can be considered for each problem when developing and evaluating a care plan.

Shortness of breath

    A primary reason for the person with COPD to enter the health-care system is usually SOB. The person may experience SOB with exertion, at rest, or intermittently, and it can have any number of causes. A thorough clinical evaluation is necessary to identify the source of the problem so that it may be dealt with effectively. Without an accurate diagnosis the results of any prescribed treatment could be minimal and possibly harmful. A number of common problems contribute to SOB:
Bronchospasm
Retained secretions
Collapsed airways (high compliance, low elasticity)
Hypoxemia
Deconditioning, ventilatory muscle fatigue
Other possibilities
    Thromboembolism
    Inhaled foreign body in the airway
    Tumor or space-occupying lesion
    Excessive extravascular fluid
    As the outline shows, the variety of conditions and anomalies that produce SOB (*source*) are tremendous. By identifying the source of the symptom, the physician and other health-care practitioners can better help the patient deal with the problem.

Once a source has been identified, treatment or therapy (*actions*) can be prescribed to alleviate the problem. Each of the different sources of a symptom may have a different treatment or combination of treatments. Therapy evaluation must be ongoing, and the health-care practitioner must be alert to changes in the patient's condition. These changes can be brought to the attention of the physician so that he can make appropriate alterations in the care plan. Some of the actions that can be taken to alleviate SOB are:

Use of a bronchodilator, in aerosol or oral form
Removal of tenacious or retained secretions
    Aerosolize bland mists
    Postural drainage, vibration/percussion
Hydration, assess fluid balance
Oxygen therapy
Relaxation techniques
Adjustment to oral medications (nonpulmonary)

Immediate relief of the primary complaint should not be the only objective of the prescribed therapy. Once the immediate crisis is under control, health-care practitioners should begin to plan the continuing care of the patient (*long-term care*). The primary element in the long-term care of the person with a chronic pulmonary disorder is education. Because the patient is likely to be returning to visit a physician over many months or even years, it is not necessary that the patient be educated in one visit. In fact, little is likely to be retained from only one presentation of material or an hour of training in self-administered therapy. Reinforcement of material should become a routine practice because the same material will need to be presented many times. Several factors should be considered throughout the months and years of a patient's treatment:

    Knowledge of the disease and its contributing factors
    Pursed-lip and diaphragmatic breathing
    Ventilation retraining
    Bronchial hygiene and relaxation
    Coordination of breathing with ADL
    Work-efficiency principles and energy conservation
    Avoidance of irritants and smoking cessation
    Indications of impending respiratory problem
    Incorporation of the family into training

The relief of the immediate problem is easily used as a sign of the effectiveness of therapy. But one must also consider the therapy over a prolonged period of time (*evaluation*). When the care plan includes criteria for evaluation, then the safety and effectiveness of therapy can be assessed. The following list suggests some of the areas to be evaluated by the health-care practitioner in optimizing respiratory care to deal with SOB:

    Medications, dose, and schedule (measurement of therapeutic blood level)

Diagnostic data, original cause for SOB
Changes in other symptoms, characteristics of patient
Breath sounds, vital signs
Somatic changes, accessory muscle use, orthopnea

Both physical and psychosocial aspects of life affect the quality of each of our lives. This is also true for the person with COPD. When developing a respiratory-care plan, the physician should not let the physical demands of the pulmonary disorder and its treatment overshadow the patient's psychologic and social needs. A comprehensive care plan should include as many aspects of life as are appropriate. Careful analysis of the patient's complaints, the therapy instituted, and medications prescribed and a history of the disorder and the patient's experience with the health-care system are important in the development of an effective care plan.

Apprehension and fear—poor coping mechanisms

There are numerous possible *sources* for the symptoms associated with the apprehension and fear of the patient and her family. Some possible sources for these symptoms are fear of death or discomfort, fear or anger over an inability to control symptoms, a poor psychosocial support network, and a lack of knowledge about the disease or prescribed therapies. This fear and anxiety can diminish the effectiveness of health care and make the patient and her family more dependent on the health-care system than necessary.

Several *actions* can be taken to relieve these symptoms or at least to reduce their effect on the overall care plan. First, in acute-care situations, do not leave the patient alone. This is especially true during situations such as severe SOB or extreme anxiety. Next, encourage the patient to vocalize concerns and fears, and be a good listener. Institute "rap" sessions, during which open discussion among concerned persons is encouraged. Once the sources of fear and anxiety have been identified, they can be dealt with more effectively, and professional help can be sought if necessary. Fears and concerns are often brought out during these discussions, helping the patient to feel less alone. Because some medications may contribute to anxiety, make sure all medications are being used correctly. Finally, the patient should learn and use relaxation exercises and other techniques to reduce and control anxiety.

Developing *long-term goals* for dealing with apprehension and fear involves considerable education and opportunities for discussion. Training for the patient and her family in relaxation techniques will take time. It may be necessary to seek professional counseling for the patient and her family or to provide opportunities for discussion of fears and concerns among family members. A discussion of the adjustments and lifestyle changes the patient and her family have experienced is important. The development of a support network of people concerned about the problems of pulmonary patients is a good long-term goal. Other pulmonary patients and the local lung association can be very valuable resources in such a support network.

When establishing the criteria for *evaluation* of fear and anxiety, the health-care practitioner should consider the patient's past coping mechanisms. It can be helpful to define the level of stress in terms of behaviors the patient can recognize and understand. For example, the patient may increase alcohol consumption or display some other habit, such as chewing on pencils or paper. Though these behaviors are not indicative of excessive stress in everyone, they may help the patient recognize her problem.

The evaluation of fear, anxiety, and other problems may require the service of a psychiatrist, psychologist, or professional counselor. This is especially true when trying to identify acute or chronic apprehension and its cause.

Somatic concerns and poor self-concept

A frequently mentioned *source* for a poor self-concept is the loss of independence that occurs in a chronic disorder. Numerous hospitalizations and traditional health care in or out of the hospital can encourage the patient to assume a dependent role. This commonly occurs in the acute-care facility but can also continue at home, at the pharmacy, or at the physician's office. Somatic concerns, stress related to finances, and altered roles within the family can also contribute to the patient's poor self-concept.

Some *actions* that may be taken to alleviate a patient's poor self-concept include a discussion of factors contributing to the problem from the patient's perspective. Attitudes about the changes in family roles and the inability to contribute, for example, income, to the family should be discussed. If financial problems are significant, a referral to a community resource such as a financial planner or credit counselor may be necessary. Psychologic counseling may be needed if severe depression is evident. A multidisciplinary *action* aspect of a care plan allows for input from a variety of resources.

The *long-term goals* for dealing with a poor self-concept can include teaching the patient to cope with a new lifestyle and recognizing the patient's assets and disabilities and the nature of her illness. During discussions, emphasis can be placed on stress reduction, relaxation, and honest encouragement of appropriate behavior. With help from the health-care practitioner, the patient should establish achievable goals, follow-up criteria, and timetables. Documentation can be designed to measure progress as well as to provide opportunities for reinforcement.

The criteria for identification and *evaluation* of a poor self-concept are often very subtle. Information such as changes in mood and mental state can be reported by reliable family members or observed by the health-care practitioner. An objective assessment of mental state can be obtained through administration of a test such as the Minnesota Multi-Phasic Personality Inventory (MMPI) or other tests recommended by a member of the mental-health team. These assessments can indicate the mental state of the patient at a given time. Observation of the interaction between the patient, her family, and the health-care staff can also be a good source of information. A positive atmosphere between the staff and the patient and her family can contribute greatly to the alleviation of a poor self-concept.

Inadequate nutrition

A number of *sources* can be suggested for the problem of poor nutrition. Some of them are anorexia, low income, fatigue, nausea from the illness or a medication, SOB (especially while eating), poor dental health, or poor dietary habits. A diary of the foods eaten over several days can be helpful in identifying problems and calculating caloric intake.

Specific dietary needs and problems are best addressed through consultation with a nutritionist. Some *actions* that can be taken to improve nutritional problems include eating frequent small meals, for example, six per day. Frequent meals can help to eliminate the feeling of fullness, which may inhibit movement of the diaphragm. The patient's family can promote a calm, pleasant, and attractive environment for eating. Meals such as casseroles or TV dinners can be planned and prepared in advance. Assistance with shopping and meal preparation can be obtained from some community organizations.

The *long-term goal* in promoting good nutrition is education. The patient and her family should be instructed to identify foods high in nutritional value. If any special needs, such as a low-salt diet, are necessary, it will be especially important to educate the patient and her family and to follow up on their implementation of dietary recommendations. Adjustments to the treatment schedule or prescribed medications may be necessary to facilitate adequate caloric and nutritional intake.

Evaluation of a patient's nutritional intake includes assessment of present dietary habits. This can be accomplished by listing the quality and quantity of food intake. A daily diary of meals, activities, and medications will also facilitate evaluation of the patient's lifestyle and its effect on nutrition. Measurement of body weight and assessment of muscle tone, skin turgor, and other physical signs can be used in the evaluation.

Low tolerance of ADL

The primary *sources* of low tolerance of ADL are SOB and apprehension. Deterioration of lung function and muscle atrophy and weakness may also make normal activities difficult. The ultimate effect of inactivity is general deconditioning. (See Chapter 5 for a discussion of the effects of inactivity.) Other problems already mentioned as common to patients with COPD, such as a reduction in energy because of poor nutrition, can also contribute to a low tolerance of ADL.

The *actions* to be taken to improve the patient's tolerance of ADL are not intended to have an immediate effect. In fact, the patient can do more harm than good by "overdoing it." It is important to resolve as many of the patient's other problems, such as poor nutrition or low self-esteem, while or even before taking action to improve her tolerance of ADL. The patient must begin a process of increasing activities and adhere to a program of reconditioning exercises over several months. Witnessing an overall improvement in the control of symptoms, the patient may be more inclined to pursue activities and maintain a level of ability.

The *long-term goals* to improve tolerance of ADL include energy conservation, reconditioning exercises, and use of techniques for increasing work efficiency. The careful scheduling of medications and activities also allows for maximum use of the patient's potential. By establishing clear, measurable, short- and long-range goals, endurance, strength, and compliance can be enhanced.

In developing criteria for *evaluation* of poor tolerance of ADL, it is important to assess the patient's functional capacity. Health-care personnel need to identify self-care problems, especially those that relate to the performance of ADL. Counseling on specific activity limits (see Appendix D) and observation and training of the patient to improve work efficiency is also important. If reasons for limits or problems are identified and explained, the patient will be more likely to adhere to recommended activities and work toward a productive lifestyle. Achievement of established goals is both a strong motivator and a good tool for evaluation.

Poor compliance with parts of the care plan

The *sources* of noncompliance with a care plan can be very complex. Some of them may be related to the patient's poor understanding of the chronic disorder and the disabilities it causes. A poor support network within the family can also limit compliance. If the patient has a poor understanding of the goals of the care program and little responsibility for the development of these goals, she will be less inclined to comply with the activities in the program.

Some *actions* that can be taken to improve compliance include ensuring that therapy is coordinated with the daily activities and routines in the patient's lifestyle. The patient should freely agree to any changes in lifestyle, which should be kept to a minimum. Follow-up visits to the physician should be regular and include clinical data to identify changes. The activity diary and all other aspects of the program should be reviewed regularly with the patient. Only essential components of the rehabilitation program should be included in the patient's home-care plan. Too much therapy done too quickly may not be well tolerated and can be discouraging.

Improving *long-term* compliance with a home-care plan must include thorough patient and family education on all aspects of the program. Particular attention should be paid to the parts of the programs that pertain to the specific complaints and problems of the patient. Emphasis should be placed on the need for patient compliance to enhance the positive outcome of the program. The patient should receive positive reinforcement when she complies with the program or when improvements are noted. The staff must maintain a positive outlook toward rehabilitation because such an attitude can be contagious.

Establishment of criteria for the *evaluation* of compliance should include family members' assessment of their participation in the program. The patient can also comment on her own efforts, both successful and futile. The correct administration of treatments, performing exercises and therapies, and taking medications should be emphasized and measured in the patient's records. A discussion between patient and staff of the level of difficulty and stress the patient experiences during activities alerts the staff to potential problems and allows for modification of the program.

THE "TEAM" CONCEPT IN LONG-TERM HEALTH CARE

Many individuals interact with and have an effect on a patient during hospitalization or other forms of medical care. Each person can make a contribution to the care of a person disabled by a pulmonary disorder. In the provision of medical care, health professionals have the largest role, as opposed to administrative personnel. But the greatest responsibility in carrying out a planned care program belongs to the patient. By involving many people in patient care, even in small ways, more opportunities for communication and reinforcement are created.

The physician is the key health-care worker involved in patient care (see Fig. 1-1). The relationship between the physician and the patient and her family can contribute significantly to the success or failure of the plan. The physician has the primary responsibility to authorize and supervise all medical care. He is also the chief provider of follow-up care, reinforcement, and encouragement. A consulting physician or specialist is often called on to assist in making the diagnosis, to recommend therapy, and to continue to evaluate the patient with a pulmonary disorder. Referral to this physician is not a transfer of the responsibility for primary care but a collaboration of sources in the development of an effective respiratory care plan.

All health-care practitioners play important roles in the development and implementation of the respiratory care plan. Each aspect of the plan should be assessed by an appropriately trained practitioner. Rehabilitation and continuing care is a multidisciplinary activity, and all available resources should be used in patient care. Good communication between the physician and the other members of the health-care team is essential to the success of the plan. This communication is important whether it takes place in an out-patient program, an in-patient program, or a home-care program or during a follow-up visit to the physician's office. Some of the reasons for and benefits of this communication are:

To allow for consistency and continuity in the quality of respiratory care

To ensure that proper, timely care is provided

To enhance the communication of changes in patient status and ideas to improve patient care

To see that all patient-care modalities fit appropriately with other aspects of the overall plan

To ensure the transmission of the physician's orders

To facilitate coordination of various aspects of care, such as timing treatment to fit in with the patient's other needs, tests, other therapy, social outlets, family, and leisure activity

Two types of health-care workers, medical and administrative, are involved with the patient and need to be included in these channels of communication. Nurses, therapists, technicians, assistants, and aides are all part of the medical section of the health-care team. Administrative support personnel also considered part of the health-care team are supervisory personnel, hospital administration, departmental management, medical records personnel, and medical social workers.

A coordinated communication effort among members of the health-care team allows for development of a well thought-out rationale for each modality ordered. It can also provide opportunities for specific assessment and application criteria for therapy and the respiratory care ordered. Such a system facilitates the physician's appraisal of patient progress or changes in patient status and, ultimately, modifications in the care provided.

COMPONENTS OF A GENERAL RESPIRATORY CARE PLAN

The respiratory care plan is made up of the following five components:
1. Problems
2. Subjective findings
3. Objective findings
4. Assessment
5. Plan

Each of these components has a number of subtopics that should be considered when writing the complete plan (Fig. 2-1). This concise, one-page format is suggested to help you organize the information.

The *problem* component of the respiratory care plan identifies specific subjects (diagnosis, complaints) to be addressed in the plan. These subjects are numbered so that subsequent components can be related to the problem the plan is intended to address. Listing problems in this manner allows the practitioner to focus on one problem at a time so that specific therapy can be mentioned to deal with the identified problem. Problems can be identified from several sources: the patient's chart, admission forms, medical history and physical examination data, and patient interview. Problems should be listed as primary (broadly categorized as pulmonary and non-pulmonary), secondary (additional problems that may or may not contribute to the primary problem), and tertiary (complaints [symptoms] to be addressed by the actions in the care plan). Listing the problems provides direction for respiratory care and overall medical care.

The *subjective findings* component of the respiratory care plan allows for input from the patient. Specific complaints and symptoms and other helpful information can be noted for consideration in developing the plan and evaluating its effectiveness. The information volunteered during the interview of the patient and family is an excellent source of such information. Open-ended questions asked during the interview can

SAMPLE FORM A

RESPIRATORY CARE PLAN for: ______________________________

DATE: ____________________

Problems or complaints:
1.
2.

Possible *sources* of problems or complaints:
1.
2.

Actions to be taken to relieve problems or complaints:
1.
2.

Goals to be achieved through actions taken:

Short-term:
1.
2.

Long-term:
1.
2.

Evaluation criteria for actions:
1.
2.

Documentation of action and follow-up required:
1.
2.

Fig. 2-1 Suggested format for organizing a respiratory care plan.

—————————————————— **SAMPLE FORM B** ——————————————————

RESPIRATORY CARE PLAN for: _____

DATE: _____

Problems:
1.
2.

Subjective findings:

Objective findings:

Assessment:

Plan:

Goals:
1.
2.

Therapeutic objectives:

Educational objectives:

Fig. 2-1 Suggested format for organizing a respiratory care plan.

OBJECTIVE DATA FOR A RESPIRATORY CARE PLAN

Physical examination

Inspection—observation of the patient
Palpation—anatomic positions and
   movements
Percussion—notes and location
Auscultation—heart and lungs (bilaterally
   [general], unilaterally [specific])

Secretions

Color
Amount
Consistency
Odor
History of occurrences of secretions and
   changes in them

Chest x-ray

P-A, interpretation
Lateral, interpretation
History of changes

Arterial blood gases

Results—pH, Pao_2, $Paco_2$, BE, Sao_2, Hb
Conditions of test, rest or exercise,
   immediately after therapy
Modes of therapy received, Fio_2

Pulmonary-function tests

Spirometry results, interpretation
Lung volumes—TLC, SVC
Other tests—DLCO, MVV, flow-volume
   loop
Exercise stress testing

Clinical lab and other laboratory findings

SMA-6, electrolytes
Sputum—culture, sensitivity, gram stain
CBC
ECG, 12 leads

---

help to identify new areas of need. Social service agencies, home health-care personnel, and health-care workers knowledgeable about the patient from previous hospitalizations can also be helpful. Some specific areas about which information should be
sought and noted in this section include:

Pain—in the chest or other areas
Sputum—color, consistency, and quantity and relation of these to past sputum produc-
   tion
Wheezing—when and where it occurs and what it is like
Dyspnea—at rest, during exertion: describe it
Effects of therapy and care in the past
Attitude/feeling toward current health status
Home remedies and medical treatments administered

There are six subparts to the *objective* component of a respiratory care plan (see box
above). The physician's examination and history is a primary source of this information. The health-care worker directly involved with the patient should confirm the
physician's findings and contribute to the data by conducting an examination and
interview of the patient. When each team member performs an assessment, especially
in his own area of expertise, the information gathered can be related to special needs
and provide a comprehensive picture of the patient's condition.

In the *assessment* component of the respiratory care plan, the health-care practitioner comments on the data gathered. This assessment is an opportunity to identify important findings and integrate them with the patient's long-term condition and needs. Specific comments can be made about the adequacy of oxygenation, Pa_{O_2}, ventilation, Pa_{CO_2}, and the removal of secretions. Conclusions drawn from the data gathered, such as the confirmation of the practitioner's findings and diagnosis, should be entered in this section. The practitioner may also add any original conclusions or observations pertinent to a specific health-care problem and any opinions or thoughts on his findings.

There are three parts to the *plan* component of the respiratory care plan:
1. *Goal* or objective to be achieved
2. *Action* or therapy to be performed
3. *Education* needed to implement therapy and resolve the short- and long-range problems associated with the disease

In a respiratory care plan, goals are broadly stated desired outcomes of the therapy to be instituted. Each goal usually pertains to the resolution of a single problem. Goals should be well thought-out, measurable, achievable, and few in number. Usually goals are long term, but they may also be short term. For example, one goal when a patient is being admitted into the hospital may be to "improve oxygenation." There is an important relationship between goals and objectives because each one plays a part in the implementation and evaluation of the care plan. For each goal there may be several objectives. When the objectives have been accomplished, the goal will have been met, and hopefully the problem will have been resolved.

Objectives in a respiratory care plan are specifically stated procedures or tasks that are related to a goal and therefore to the identified problem. They are often sequential steps directed at the accomplishment of a particular goal. Many objectives may be required to accomplish one goal. Objectives may contain statements for judging effectiveness or criteria for monitoring accomplishment of a goal, such as "O_2 at 2 L/ min by cannula, monitor Sa_{O_2} with ear oximeter and maintain $Sa_{O_2} > 85\%$ at rest." Most frequently the objectives in a respiratory care plan will be specific to pulmonary problems, such as weaning parameters and extubation criteria. Occasionally goals and objectives may be needed to address problems not directly related to the pulmonary disorder, such as muscle fatigue caused by poor nutrition or decubitus caused by poor mobility. If the person writing the care plan identifies a problem outside her area of expertise, she should seek assistance from qualified professionals in that field.

Both short- and long-range goals for the patient should be considered when writing the care plan. Short-term goals are directed at the immediate problems that have been identified. They also ensure that any acute symptoms are quickly controlled, preventing further complications. Short-term goals and their accompanying objectives provide direction for performance and assessment of daily therapy and care.

Long-range goals ensure that chronic problems, which may be considered a "given" in a pulmonary disorder, are not ignored while immediate needs are cared for. These goals provide a guide for care while treatment is progressing toward the eventual discharge of the patient and allow the practitioner to maintain a perspective on the many abnormal physical conditions that may exist in a patient. A long-term goal also provides a standard by which to judge the effects of therapies and procedures in the care plan. It may be that the "normal" state for a patient includes wheezing upon exhalation or sputum production upon coughing. If this is true, then it may be inappropriate to attempt to clear the chest of all adventitious breath sounds or cure the cough. If the patient complains of fewer symptoms than she did before therapy was implemented, the practitioner can consider the reduction a good indication of progress. Long-term goals also allow for consideration of the lifestyle of the patient in the development of a long-term plan. It may become apparent once the patient's lifestyle is considered that established goals are inappropriate. For example, the ability to walk to the mailbox may be just as satisfying to the patient as a walk around the block. Or it may be that the patient has domestic help in her home and does not need to be concerned with housekeeping chores as was first believed. When a "normal" state for the patient has been identified and all variables in the patient's lifestyle have been considered, the staff and the patient can measure changes, and the plan can be individualized to better meet the needs of the patient and her family.

"Actions or Therapeutic Interventions" is a list of each therapy to be administered to the patient. These therapies are written out as completely as possible by the health-care practitioner. This order should mention any necessary coordination with other care being given to the patient. To maximize the effectiveness of therapy, the patient's special needs should be considered, for example, limited mobility of the patient's leg caused by arthritis, manual ventilation to hyperinflate the patient's lungs or measurement of the volume of inhalation during each aerosol treatment, and administration of oxygen only during ambulation. Any therapy that is prescribed should adhere to established limits to allow the practitioner to assess the effectiveness of treatment.

Education in a care plan should include an explanation to the patient and her family of the therapies currently being administered. The purpose, method, and duration of treatment should be clarified. Potential questions about topics such as the function of an endotracheal or a tracheostomy tube, the need for communication and how to communicate with an intubated patient, the purpose of aerosol therapy, and the name and effects of medications should be addressed. All treatments and therapies should be explained, and questions should be encouraged to allow the patient and family to participate in the administration of the therapy. The anatomy and pathophysiology of the patient's disease and the equipment, procedures, and medications that will be used to treat that illness will need to be explained. This early communication will be greatly beneficial to future communication with the patient and family. Ultimately suggestions can be made for any rehabilitation or education that will be necessary to implement the revised care plan developed when the patient is discharged. Reinforcement of self-care techniques and healthy lifestyle habits and instruction on handling emergencies and recognizing warning signs of impending problems may be necessary.

The criteria for judging the effectiveness and subsequently the continuation of each therapy in a respiratory care plan should be clearly established and written. The most obvious indication to discontinue therapy is the absence of any indications for treatment. For example, in oxygenation an adequate Pao_2 on room air may be a criterion for ending treatment. In postural drainage the absence of productive sputum coughing for 48 hours may indicate termination of treatment. In bland aerosol therapy adequate hydration may be indicated by skin turgor and the diminished viscosity of secretions, and this would be a sufficient basis for discontinuing treatment. It may be that the original problem for which the patient required treatment has been resolved. This resolution can be indicated by the successful withdrawal of treatment mechanisms, such as a chest tube, or by the patient's independent demonstration of skills, such as ambulation. Finally, patient treatment may reach a point at which it automatically stops, for example, if it has been designed to stop after 5 days. At this point the patient's condition and treatment should automatically be assessed before a decision is made to continue, change, or discontinue a treatment.

Collecting data from a patient

It is extremely important to establish rapport between the patient and the staff of a rehabilitation or home-care program. Helping the patient cope with the problems associated with her disease requires an understanding and appreciation of the patient's point of view. By responding to the person from her frame of reference and by not forcing artificial conditions on her, the health-care practitioner can reinforce the patient's sense of self-worth. Open communication with the patient about her concerns creates an atmosphere in which the health-care practitioner can share from his own experience and expertise effective ways to deal with the patient's problems. A goal in helping any patient should be to give her the opportunity to change behaviors and develop effective mechanisms for coping with her own disability. An open, cooperative relationship between the patient and the health-care practitioner is the first step toward this goal.

The foundation for a good relationship is set during the practitioner's earliest interview with the patient and her family. The roles that each person involved with the rehabilitation process will assume are established early (first impressions count) and can be difficult to change later. It will be important to identify persons the patient can relate to and communicate with. At times a particular staff or family member will be able to communicate most effectively with the patient. This person should serve as the conduit for important information to and from the patient. As the patient progresses through the rehabilitation program, additional persons can become more involved. Perhaps the hospital nutritionist or pharmacist or one of the therapists or technicians may be able to communicate best with the patient. Opportunities for all staff to interact and develop a relationship with the patient should be encouraged. Because of limited or sporadic contact with the patient, some staff members may have to make a special effort to develop this relationship.

It is likely that the patient will have been interviewed many times by the time she is ready for a rehabilitation program. In order not to elicit standard answers from the patient, frank and open communication is necessary. The staff's attitude should be that rehabilitation is a new beginning for the patient and that the patient's feelings and opinions are important. The information gathered from one pulmonary patient usually will not be different from information obtained from any other pulmonary patient, but each individual's perceptions and coping behaviors will be different. Recognizing these differences can be critical in maximizing the effectiveness of program activities. Once a patient is part of the health-care system, she is usually encouraged to play a passive, dependent role. But passiveness and dependence are not what members of the rehabilitation staff want, and they should work during their initial contacts with the patient to prevent these traits from developing. It is important to cover all areas of concern thoroughly during an interview. The staff should allow time during the interview for the patient to ask questions and to share incidents that she feels will better communicate her situation and experiences.

At the beginning of the interview the health-care practitioner should introduce himself and any other staff members present. He should state the purpose for his presence and the presence of anyone with him and obtain permission from the patient to proceed with the interview. The atmosphere during the interview should be comfortable, relaxed, and unhurried. Staff members should project the attitude that they are entering the patient's private domain so that the patient gets the feeling of having some control. Because some points may be brought up again later for clarification or discussion, the interviewer should take notes on what is said and done during the interview.

Professionalism in requesting information is imperative. All questions and topics brought up during the interview should be expressed in the same objective tone and with the same objective attitude. This objectivity will be especially important when areas of particular sensitivity to the patient are being discussed. But the staff should avoid presuming that a certain topic is sensitive and will be difficult for the patient to discuss because such presumptions are often incorrect. Tactful questioning and consideration for individual rights are interview skills that are acquired with experience, so interviewers should take every opportunity to practice them.

Asking questions

Writing and asking a good question for an interview is not an easy task. For example, it is important that the interviewer not lead the patient to any standard answers. A patient being interviewed often can sense when a positive or negative answer is expected. The patient may supply only the expected answer when she would have preferred to elaborate on it or to qualify the response to make it *her* answer based on *her* experiences. Questions that can be answered with *yes* or *no* are not desirable in an interview because a simple *yes* or *no* answer does not supply much information. On the other hand, open questions, which can usually begin with the words *who, what, when, where, why,* and *how,* allow the patient to fill in all of the necessary information. Questions should not be forced into an open-question format, but with practice most of them can be expressed this way. Asking questions in this manner allows the patient to provide the information the rehabilitation staff is seeking in her own words and from her own perspective.

Openness during an interview is created by several factors, including the type of questions and the manner in which they are asked, the position in the room of the patient in relation to the interviewer, the presence of family members and staff, and the climate in the room. Nonverbal communication, such as body position, facial expression, and eye contact can be a valuable source of information. Failure to be sensitive to these and other factors can impair the free exchange of information during an interview. The person doing the interview needs to establish his credibility and affirm his right to ask questions. Job titles, degrees, or permission forms from a physician are not all that is needed to establish the interviewer's right to ask questions. Sharing personal or professional experiences in the area of pulmonary disease is a good way to gain the patient's confidence. The staff's openness often encourages openness from the patient being interviewed.

Listening

The reason for asking a question is to listen to the response. If the reason for asking were merely to receive information, then words alone would be adequate. But effective listening is a skill that begins with having a reason to listen and knowing what to listen for in the words and tone of a response.

The interviewer's nonverbal communication can have a significant effect on the quality and quantity of information discussed during an interview. With his legs and arms uncrossed, the interviewer should sit in a way that suggests a receptive attitude. He should look at the patient being interviewed, at least while the patient is answering a question, but not in an intimidating or judgmental manner. The interviewer's facial expressions should indicate concentration, enthusiasm, and anticipation of information. Perhaps the most difficult aspect of listening is ignoring distractions, a necessary requirement for a successful interview. The interviewer should position himself in the room to minimize distractions and face the patient being interviewed.

Although the interviewer wants the patient to feel free to share anything she feels is important, he must also keep her on the subject. This can be difficult with a talkative patient or family member but can be accomplished by referring back to the form being used to record information.

It is best to record information from the interview in an orderly format that is

```
┌─ SUGGESTED TOPIC AREAS TO COVER DURING A PATIENT INTERVIEW ─┐
```

Primary symptom

Symptoms (coughing, sputum production, wheezing, and SOB, given in order of onset

Personal history

Background, living habits, environment
Socioeconomic status, past and present
Cigarette abuse, past and present
Character of typical chest cold
Any kind of chest illness or other past illness

Family history

Serious illness or deaths in immediate family
Patient's previous illnesses and treatments

Occupational history
(Organize chronologically.)

Types of jobs the patient has held
Conditions in the patient's workplace

familiar to the program staff. Such a format allows everyone who reads the information to locate quickly what they wish to know. It can also reduce the need for patient and family to repeat the same information to several individuals. The box above suggests broad topics to cover when interviewing a patient and her family. (Appendix A includes a format for recording interview information, a sequence to follow during an interview, and suggested questions in each topic area.)

BIBLIOGRAPHY

Ahmad M and Lindquist C: Bronchial asthma: some aspects of pathogenesis and therapy, Postgrad Med 62(1):111-118, 1977.

Bartlett RH et al: Respiratory maneuvers to prevent postoperative pulmonary complications, JAMA 224(7): 1017-1021, 1973.

Benjamin SP and McCormack LT: Structural abnormalities in COPD, Postgrad Med 62(1):101-106, 1977.

Buckingham WR: Diagnosing chronic obstructive pulmonary disease, Mod Med 46(2):53-61, 1978.

Cherniack RM et al: Breathing easy: a panel discussion, Emerg Med 27-45, Dec 1977.

Cordasco EM and VanOrdstrand HS: Air pollution and COPD, Postgrad Med 62(1):124-127, 1977.

Fergus LC and Cordasco EM: Pulmonary rehabilitation of the patient with COPD, Postgrad Med 62(1): 141-144, 1977.

Gaensler EA and Wright GW: Evaluation of respiratory impairment, Arch Environ Health 12:146-189, Feb 1966.

Golish JA and Ahmad M: Management of COPD: a physiologic approach, Postgrad Med 62(1):131-136, 1977.

Hodgkin JE, editor: Chronic obstructive pulmonary disease: current concepts in diagnosis and comprehensive care, 1979, American College of Chest Physicians.

Hodgkin JE, Zorn E, and Connors G: Pulmonary rehabilitation: guidelines to success, Stoneham, Mass, 1984, Butterworth Publishers.

Mathers J, Cooper K, and Glauser F: Office management of COPD, Geriatrics 36(1):103-111, 1981.

Robbins JA and Mushlin AI: Preoperative evaluation of the healthy patient, Med Clin North Am 63(6): 1145-1156, 1979.

Tomashefski JF: Definition, differentiation, and classification of COPD, Postgrad Med 62(1):88-97, 1977.

CHAPTER 3

Patient and family education in rehabilitation and home care

EDUCATION AND REHABILITATION

A major objective of long-term care of the patient with COPD is modification of behaviors and habits to optimize the patient's ability to function in a way as normal as possible. The health-care practitioner involved with the pulmonary patient must help to build the patient's self-reliance and sense of responsibility for his own health care. When a patient with a pulmonary disorder understands the disease, the intent of the therapy described, and the expected outcomes of therapy, he builds a solid foundation for incorporating therapy into his daily activities. The patient needs to recognize that he can prevent further lung damage and that much can be done to improve the disabling effects of the pulmonary disorder. By clearly identifying which aspects of the disease are reversible and which are not, patient compliance can be improved. The key to the success of long-term care is increased patient confidence in his own ability to administer self-care correctly, to recognize changes in his condition, and to communicate with the other members of his health-care team.

Family members and other people in the patient's support network should be integral parts of the education process. The most significant person in the patient's relationships should be identified and included in the education program whenever possible. Though family members should not perform all the therapy involved in the continuing care of the patient, they can help by making the patient accountable for his own care. During exacerbations of the illness, a family member's opinion can often affect decisions that are made based on objective findings in a patient. For example, a change in the quantity or color of sputum produced or in the patient's demeanor or daily activities can be corroborated by a family member.

Patient/family education, as used in this context, means primarily the transmittal

Table 3-1 Differences between education and rehabilitation

	Patient/family education	Pulmonary rehabilitation
Objectives	Short-term	Long-term
Primary function	To transmit information	To modify behavior and lifestyle habits

of information from one source to another. Cognitive material, knowledge, and psychomotor skills make up the material presented to the patient and his family. It is imperative that only essential facts and skills be presented because too much material presented in too rapid a manner or over a short period of time can contribute to poor compliance. However, it is important to realize that facts, procedures, and affective content, such as attitudes, in a patient-education program will not change behavior by themselves. Knowledge alone does not change behavior. For example, a large number of people continue to smoke even though the evidence is conclusive that smoking damages health. It is important to recognize from the beginning that a patient-education program is not directed solely at behavior modification though it may be hoped that a behavior change will result from the new information provided to the patient and his family. The intent of an education program is to put the necessary knowledge for understanding the disability and what is being done about it into the patient's hands (Table 3-1).

Studies of education and retention have demonstrated that only 10% to 20% of new material presented to an individual one time is retained for an extended period of time, such as more than a year. If the individual uses the material, retention can be greater than 50%. The educational component of a health-care program should be constructed to include built-in repetition and application of important material. The health-care practitioner teaching the patient will find the task much easier if specific lesson plans are designed, handouts are organized, and forms are patient-oriented and simple. It should also be understood that one session on the patient's pulmonary disease and disability generally will not be sufficient to educate the individual on that topic. Multiple sessions should be scheduled at times and places to optimize the learning process. The patient and family must be aware of the objectives of each lesson and the importance of the material to their medical problems and other needs. A formal educational session should last about 20 minutes, and several sessions in a single day would be far more beneficial than one long lecture or demonstration. If the material is too voluminous, it should be broken down into manageable segments.

Once the patient has been introduced to the educator and understands that the physician supports the education program, learning sessions can begin. The sequence of events during a lesson may be as follows:
1. Introduce the topic.
2. State objectives (the intended outcome for the patient).
3. Present the material in sequence with the objectives.

4. Restate what the patient should now know (according to the objectives).
5. Answer questions and "personalize" the content.
6. "Quiz" the patient on the material to reinforce major points.

A subsequent session with the patient can begin with a quick review of the previously covered material for reinforcement and for correction of any of the patient's misunderstandings. This session also allows the new material to be related to the previous material so that the information does not seem out of context.

The patient with a chronic lung disease generally learns a great deal about health care during his hospital stay. Some of what is learned is not always helpful for the patient's long-term care. For example, the patient often learns that he can assume a dependent, passive role in the hospital—one that is opposite of the role he will be required to assume upon discharge. But both the patient and the hospital staff should remember that the patient may have to perform at home some of the therapy provided in the hospital. The consistency of hospital care and the attitude of the health-care practitioner demonstrate to the patient the importance of treatments and therapies being administered. The quality of this hospital care and the hospital staff's attention to detail become the standard against which the patient and his family will measure how well they should perform the same therapy at home.

This means that everyone who comes into contact with a patient in the hospital affects the process of educating that patient. Information the patient will need to perform self-care should be reinforced at every opportunity. The patient should be encouraged to ask questions and to assume responsibility for the various facets of self-care, for example, taking medications on a regular schedule. For each medication the patient should know (1) the name, (2) the reason for prescription, (3) the method of administration, (4) the schedule of administration, and (5) the side effects. Keeping in mind the six steps to be followed during an educational session (p. 42), the health-care practitioner can communicate this information each time a medication is administered. It is possible for the practitioner to transmit a great deal of information to a patient and his family during the sometimes numerous days of a patient's hospitalization.

The education process begins when the patient is admitted into the hospital, although at the time he may not be able to participate in a significant way by devoting attention to the process or performing a task. It is important to begin soon after admission to build the patient's attitude that he will be going home eventually and will be responsible for carrying out the care plan. The patient's loss of independence alone can be very debilitating and depressing even without taking into account the physical problems associated with the disease. For the patient in an intensive care unit (ICU) the amount of independence he will be able to display certainly will be minimal.

Communication and the building of trust in health-care practitioners also begins upon admission, and the long-term effects of education should be kept in mind even at such an early stage of care. Many patients do not distinguish well among doctors, nurses, therapists, technicians, and other people wearing a uniform in the hospital,

┌──┐

— POINTS TO EMPHASIZE DURING PATIENT AND FAMILY EDUCATION —

1. The significance of the results of pulmonary-function tests, such as FEV_1, FEF_{25-75}, and RV/TLC ratio, especially if these tests will be repeated, to evaluate progression or improvement of lung condition. It should be emphasized that an obstructive pulmonary disorder makes it difficult to get air out of the lungs, as opposed to a restrictive disorder, in which it is difficult to get air into the lungs or a pulmonary vascular disorder, which may also cause dyspnea.
2. Which effects of the disease are reversible and which are not. Alveolar damage, loss of surface area as demonstrated by a decrease in the DLCO, is not reversible. However, bronchospasm, inflammation of the airways, and excess secretions can be reversed.
3. Any changes in the patient's lifestyle that can prevent further damage to the lungs. Smoking is the chief contributor to pulmonary malfunction. Occupational hazards and the patient's home environment and lifestyle habits must also be considered.
4. The patient should understand what his pulmonary disorder is *not*. Cancer, tuberculosis, and heart disease may have been ruled out through testing. The patient needs to understand that these problems are not associated with the lung disorder.

└──┘

and every health-care practitioner affects the education of the patient and contributes to his well-being. Both structured (formal) and unstructured (informal) teaching can be effective ways of transmitting information to the patient. Each staff member should be ready to give answers to the patient's questions or be willing to direct the questions to someone who can answer them. Interpersonal relationships with the staff are a key element in patient education and improved compliance with prescribed therapy.

ASSESSING READINESS TO LEARN

Once a formal program of patient education is to begin, the attitude of the patient and family toward the process must be assessed. A patient who has recently been informed that he has a chronic disease, such as emphysema, may not be able to cope immediately with the disorder and its accompanying disabilities. The patient must deal with this information by going through stages similar to the stages involved in the resolution of a major life crisis, such as a death. The steps in the process of mentally and emotionally dealing with the disease and its accompanying lifestyle changes are (1) shock, grief, and sometimes anger, (2) denial, (3) acknowledgement and acceptance, and (4) adaptation. The patient must progress through all of these steps to reach the healthiest and most constructive outlook on his condition.

The patient and his family should keep in mind that the patient will not progress through all of these steps simultaneously. Frequently the process is repeated when the patient receives new information. Once the stage the patient is at is identified, patient-education techniques and information can be individualized. Although the fourth step, adaptation, is the healthiest and most conducive to learning, the patient in the hospital is not often at this point. More time is needed for the individual to "work through" his grief than is generally spent in the hospital resolving the acute aspects of the illness. The health-care practitioner's willingness to answer questions and talk openly and honestly about the disorder can be very helpful to the patient during this difficult time. Frequently the practitioner must give the patient information while he is not ready to deal with it. This is usually done with the hope that the patient will recall the information and find it useful at a time when he is coping with the disease better.

A patient in the second stage, denial, is the most difficult to teach. At this point the physician's input and sometimes professional counseling can enable the patient to cope more effectively with the disease. Support and care from the health-care team encourage the patient to accept the diagnosis and maintain channels of communication for future patient education.

Society today contributes to the attitude that there is a "cure" or a quick solution for every problem. Understanding and coping with the reality that there is no "cure" for his disease may be very difficult for the patient. It is important for the patient to understand as many facts as possible about his condition. To facilitate understanding, the practitioner should perform and thoroughly explain to the patient pulmonary function studies and any other diagnostic tests or procedures, such as bronchoscopy or exercise testing. Points that should be emphasized during patient and family education are given in the box on p. 42.

The practitioner should keep in mind that often the patient and the family are not initially prepared for the psychologic and emotional changes brought about by the identification of a pulmonary problem. The initial information about the disease should be communicated in positive form. During early education sessions the practitioner should reinforce the patient's self-worth and assure the patient and his family that they can do a great deal to maintain and improve their lifestyle. It is no longer acceptable merely to tell the patient to go home, minimize physical exertion, and avoid people with colds.

It is important that the relationship between the physician and the patient be respected as the primary source of the patient's positive attitude toward his disability. The physician's positive attitude toward the education process increases the patient's willingness to participate. The physician should be involved with patient and family education from the beginning. The physician should also have an intimate knowledge of the components of any therapeutic program designed for the patient's home use. Obviously she is aware of the medications and oxygen being administered to the patient because she prescribed them, but frequently she may not be aware of the educational needs and rehabilitative aspects of a home-care program.

APTITUDE OF THE PATIENT AND THE FAMILY

Some patients have no mechanical aptitude and have demonstrated an extreme lack of skill in performance of routine psychomotor activities. This does not mean that an individual is not intelligent or able to understand the desired procedure. But many times it may be extremely difficult for the patient or his family to use some machines, implement treatments, and follow schedules when they are not used to a routine or to using tools.

An assessment of the psychomotor skills of the patient and his family should be made as part of the initial patient evaluation. Often the person who does most of the cooking in the home is used to dealing with various utensils and therefore uses psychomotor skills regularly. If this person is not the patient, other activities that develop psychomotor skills can be used as starting points for teaching these skills. By relating skills involved in the prescribed therapy to tasks familiar to the patient, the health-care practitioner can help the patient to understand new skills better. For example, someone who cooks regularly will be very familiar with measuring in teaspoons, tablespoons, and cups but may be unfamiliar with weights, volumes, and lengths when used in a different context. A person who has changed the oil in a car can understand measurements such as quarts and liters and movements such as turning an object clockwise and counterclockwise. This experience can provide familiar comparisons for understanding medication volume and equipment assembly. One family member may be responsible for mixing or preparing the individual doses of the patient's medications. This can be done ahead of time, and the small quantities can be stored in the refrigerator. With the help of these premeasured medication doses, the patient is able to administer his own treatment, maintaining some control over his own health care.

PLANNING A LESSON

Standardized content of patient education in COPD promotes consistency in patient information and eliminates confusion and frustration for the entire health-care team. Communication among health-care practitioners about the content of patient education and the roles each practitioner should play enhances the education process. It is best if one individual has primary responsibility for patient education. Ideally this person would be the patient's physician, but it is not realistic to expect from the physician the tremendous time commitment required to teach the patient and his family all they need to know about the disease and about caring for their needs. It is important that the physician support the education process and agree with the content being presented. By determining the content of a patient-education program, developing its objectives and handouts, and communicating its organization to the other members of the health-care team, the physician can ensure continuity of care and improve patient education.

COMMON MISCONCEPTIONS ABOUT OXYGEN THERAPY

Oxygen is addictive.
If a little oxygen is good, more is better.
SOB is always caused by lack of oxygen.
A patient receiving oxygen therapy is confined to the home.
Oxygen will burn and is explosive.

SAMPLE MATERIAL FOR PATIENT EDUCATION

Following is sample material from which to draw a lesson plan on oxygen therapy for patient and family education. This material can serve as a beginning point, but specific information about the patient's condition and medications and the equipment necessary for treatment would need to be emphasized in other lessons. Sample lesson plans are given at the end of the chapter.

Five common misconceptions about oxygen therapy are given in the box above. Correcting or clarifying these five points could be the objective of a lesson in oxygen therapy because it is important that the patient and his family have a clear understanding of oxygen and its use in the home.

Although it is necessary for life, oxygen is *not* an addictive substance. On the other hand, nicotine and morphine are two well-known addictive substances and are listed by the World Health Organization (WHO) as such. But oxygen does not meet the WHO's criteria for addictive substances. Some patients receiving oxygen therapy may experience an improvement in their pulmonary condition and be able to decrease or even eliminate the use of oxygen therapy, which would not be possible if oxygen were addictive.

Too much oxygen can be just as harmful as too little oxygen, a fact that has been known for some time. Antoine LaVoisier, a French physician and chemist, experimented in the late 1700s with mice and reported that too much or too little oxygen caused them to die. Oxygen is a gas that is prescribed by flow rate, a number of liters of gas per minute. A patient receiving oxygen therapy may believe that if he increases the prescribed flow rate for oxygen during an episode of SOB, he will be less uncomfortable. This may not be the case, so the flow rate should be changed only on the order of a physician.

SOB is not always caused by a lack of oxygen in the blood. For example, people with normal lungs and pulmonary function feel short of breath when their pulmonary muscles are fatigued after extreme exertion, such as when a football player runs 100 yards for a touchdown. A patient with a pulmonary disorder who does not have heart disease may also experience SOB, for example, when taking a walk, that is not caused by a need for an increased oxygen-flow rate. The oxygen in the blood is most likely within its normal range, so in this case oxygen therapy would not be beneficial. Instead the patient needs rest. The only way to be sure oxygen is needed is to measure the amount of oxygen in the blood during particular situations or activities. (See also the desaturation study in Chapter 5.)

When oxygen is indicated and an oxygen system is selected, the patient's lifestyle and interests should be considered. The patient on oxygen therapy is not confined to the home. Technologic advances in oxygen-therapy equipment have made traveling with the equipment much more manageable than it once was. Patients receiving oxygen therapy at home can travel, go out to dinner, and participate in most of the normal activities of life. At times special arrangements must be made for car, air, and sea travel, but the equipment company can help with these arrangements. Shopping and visiting should be encouraged.

Another major misunderstanding about oxygen therapy is that oxygen is flammable and explosive. Oxygen is neither flammable nor explosive. Oxygen supports combustion: an object cannot burn if oxygen is not present, and a fire is more likely to start when oxygen in an enclosed space is at higher levels than normal. But the gas itself does not burn. The belief in the explosiveness of oxygen comes from the few instances of a cylinder under high pressure (2000 psig) breaking open and rapidly, "explosively," releasing the gas. For example, if a cylinder of oxygen were knocked over and the valve were broken, the released pressure could drive a cylinder through a wall. Cylinders should be secure, and smoking, heat, and open flames should be kept away from areas in which oxygen is being used. These precautions should be taken not because oxygen will burn or explode but because any material that will burn will do so much more quickly in the presence of oxygen.

CURRICULUM DEVELOPMENT AND TOPICS IN PATIENT EDUCATION

Lesson plans should be developed for each content area to be included in the curriculum for patient and family education. Some of the topics to be addressed are given in the box on p. 47. The areas should be broken further into discrete topics to be covered at each lesson. (Additional topics and details for each content area can be found in Appendix B. Some sample lesson plans are given at the end of this chapter.) It is important to have a goal in mind for each formal education session. The objectives for each lesson should relate to the goal and must be measurable. The patient and the instructor must be able to recognize when the objective has been accomplished. Descriptive behavioral terms can be helpful when writing the objectives for a lesson. Each objective should be one sentence long and can start with terms such as *name, explain, demonstrate, describe, identify, assemble, calculate,* or *draw.* These written objectives keep each session on focus. Written lesson plans also show the patient and the instructor the direction in which treatment is going and how far it has progressed and allow for the measurement of results.

_____ **TOPICS FOR EDUCATING THE PATIENT WITH COPD** _____

Pulmonary anatomy and physiology
COPD—pathophysiology, diagnostic tests, and contributing factors
Manifestations, symptoms, and progression of COPD
Medications and other therapeutic treatments
Nutrition and hydration
Smoking cessation
Control of environment and avoidance of infection
ADL, energy conservation
Warning signs of infection and when to seek help
Retraining in diaphragmatic and pursed-lip breathing
Breathing exercises, ventilation retraining for activity
Therapeutic treatments
Operating, caring for, and cleaning respiratory equipment
Strength and endurance training
Relaxation training
Pulmonary terminology, roles of health-care providers
Community resources for COPD patients
Record keeping, personal health care
Insurance and third-party reimbursement

The patient and family should be aware of the objectives for each lesson and have some input into their development. They should know how treatment is progressing and what their strengths and weaknesses as part of the treatment process are. Input from the patient and family, especially about how they will accomplish tasks at home, should be encouraged. The time devoted to education should allow for discussion of the patient and family's feelings about the disease and its treatment and of the patient's feelings about his disease and disabilities. This discussion allows the patient and his family to contribute to their own understanding of each lesson and to apply it to their own lives.

Because explaining to the patient the many topics to be covered in an education program when it begins may overwhelm the patient and make coping with the disease even more difficult, it is best to explain merely that a number of topics will be discussed and to give details during individual lessons or as the patient and family request them. Because the patient usually wants to know, the end of a program should be clearly identified. A method of evaluating the patient's progress relative to the goals and objectives of the program must be discussed and be agreed upon by both the instructor and the patient. A question-and-answer session is one method. A discussion of any change in symptoms or abilities as noted by the patient, family, or instructor is another method. Mastery of a psychomotor skill and even a paper-and-pencil test are other alternatives. A feeling of accomplishment should accompany the completion of each segment of a program. Periodic evaluation provides objective evidence of progress and, along with positive verbal comments from the instructor, improves compliance and self-esteem tremendously.

The goals of in-patient education differ from those of a rehabilitation program. Patient-education goals must be short-term and focused primarily on transmitting information. Effective information transmission generally means writing objectives in relatively low-level terms: *list, name, describe,* or *demonstrate* specific skills. Changes in behavior require a more intensive approach and certainly more time than is usually allowed for patient education alone. A patient-education program should not aim to modify the patient's lifestyle and habits. Although it is possible that these changes will occur, education alone generally will not change behavior. A typical means of demonstrating learning is the ability of the learner to repeat, without supervision, the behavior being taught. When a patient takes information and incorporates it into behavior, he possesses the additional asset of being able to teach himself.

Follow-up after discharge from the hospital or completion of an education program is an integral part of the education process because it allows for reinforcement of the values and other material being taught to the patient. Follow-up can be in many forms, such as a letter from the instructor, a phone call from a health-care practitioner who provided care, or a visit from a social worker or from a representative of the home care–equipment provider. Each follow-up method has strengths and weaknesses, but the important point is that the patient continues to be monitored in some way. Follow-up allows for fine tuning of the patient's home-care program. Some parts of the program may be working while others are not. Perhaps the patient is having difficulty in a particular situation because he forgot to ask a question about it. If such difficulties are not resolved, the patient's compliance with the medical program will diminish. Many patients also have a feeling of isolation and often do not feel that they are truly part of their health-care team. Perhaps the best method of follow-up is a visit to the physician's office, which gets the patient involved in his own care more than any other method and keeps the physician informed about the patient's condition. The physician can also emphasize the parts of the home-care program that are most important for the patient's therapy regimen. An encouraging word from the physician and reinforcement of the material taught in the education program can boost the patient's confidence.

Each patient should be treated as an individual; each one's priorities and perception of needs should influence the type of patient-education material chosen and the manner in which it is presented. It is difficult to assess a patient's readiness and ability to learn and motivation to comply with a program of self-care. As health-care providers, we should never accept full responsibility for the long-term care of the patient. We should accept responsibility in the acute-care setting, but our minds should always be on preparing the patient and his family for the continuation of care. The measure of the success of a hospitalization should not be discharging the patient but preventing his return because of an exacerbation of the illness.

SUGGESTIONS FOR EFFECTIVE TEACHING

The suggestions for instructors given in the box below have been found to be helpful in improving teaching. Many of them are merely common sense. By checking herself against these guidelines from time to time, an instructor can make sure she is giving her best effort to the lesson and the patient.

SUGGESTIONS TO IMPROVE TEACHING

Be prepared. Show commitment to the patient's education and to the value of the content of the lesson. Have all materials necessary for the lesson on hand. If a question was asked in the last session that you were unable to answer, be sure to have the answer at the next session.

Be organized. Follow the plan as written. Keep the objectives in mind and demonstrate progression through the material at every opportunity.

Be flexible. Allow the patient to have input into his education. Alter the planned objectives or sequence of topics to allow for momentary deviations. Structure in an education plan should be a framework within which to work, not the goal of the effort.

Include questions in presentations. The patient will not learn the material if he is not involved in the education process. Encourage the patient to ask questions, and ask him to explain what has been said in his own words.

Say it, demonstrate it, have the patient do it, and then practice it. Telling is not teaching. By following these steps the patient becomes involved immediately. Corrections can be made before mistakes become imbedded in the patient's mind, and positive reinforcement can be given for correct answers or behavior. A patient learns through what he does, not through what the instructor does or says.

Avoid jargon. Do not talk down to the patient or assume that he knows what is meant. Make a habit of explaining words that cannot be avoided and avoiding words that will only complicate the material. Generally these are words outside the immediate subject area that require digression from the main topic to explain them.

Show enthusiasm. A positive attitude is contagious, and enthusiasm for the patient's potential is encouraging to the patient. Let him know that he may experience setbacks and that the skills to be learned are not easy but that the emphasis is on improvement.

Use audiovisual aids. Audiovisual aids (AV) are helpful, especially when used during a lesson. However, AV aids should not be used as substitutes for the instructor's preparation and knowledge.

Encourage personalization of the material. Group lessons are effective for transmitting basic information, but to ensure the individual patient has understood the essential points, the instructor should provide one-on-one lessons. Open discussion of basic material provides a safe social outlet, and frequently other patients are the most effective teachers. Be sure the patient can internalize the material and can think of one application or implication for each lesson.

SAMPLE LESSON PLANS FOR TOPICS IN COPD EDUCATION
Topic: nutrition and hydration

Upon completion of this unit, the patient and his family should be able to:
1. Name the six essential nutrients in a balanced diet
2. Name one type of food he likes that is a source of one or more of the six essential nutrients
3. Name three things that can be done to eliminate a bloated feeling or abdominal distension, which hamper breathing
4. Describe how dry milk can be used to increase the nutritional value of food
5. List the types of fluids that can be included to ensure adequate hydration and list the fluids to be avoided
6. List the amount of fluid that should be consumed on a daily basis when on a program of hydration
7. Name two signs that indicate that the patient needs more fluids
8. List four foods high in potassium, which should be consumed when the patient is taking diuretics
9. Describe two ways to improve the patient's appetite at meal times
10. Identify the patient's normal weight

Topic: the warning signs of infection and when to seek help for an infection

Upon completion of this unit, the patient and his family should be able to:
1. List the major symptoms that characterize the patient's "normal" disease state, such as cough, sputum production, sputum color, sensation of breathlessness, body condition and color, condition of ankles, skin pinch, sleep habits, and wheezing
2. Name three specific changes that should be brought to the attention of the physician as soon as they are noticed
3. Give the patient's normal oral body temperature
4. Describe a network of contacts to be made in the event of an emergency and write out the names and phone numbers of the people to be contacted
5. Discriminate a true emergency from a change in symptoms and describe an emergency situation
6. Describe the changes in the patient's "normal" disease state that may indicate the presence of an infection
7. Describe the self-care procedure to be followed when the patient experiences an increase in wheezing or SOB

Topic: medications

Upon completion of this unit, the patient and his family should be able to:

1. Explain the difference between generic and brand-name drugs
2. List each medication the patient is taking and the dosage
3. Describe the action of each medication
4. Define "side effect"
5. Describe the physical appearance of each medication
6. List on a daily schedule the times when each medication should be taken
7. Name any special precautions or procedures for taking medications
8. Demonstrate the proper technique for inhalation from a metered-dose device
9. Describe how to measure the contents of a metered-dose device
10. Describe the possible side effects of each medication

BIBLIOGRAPHY

Bille DA: A study of patient's knowledge in relation to teaching format and compliance, Supervisor Nurse 55-62, March 1977.

Blue Cross Association: White paper: patient health education, Atlanta, Aug 1974, Health Care Services.

Branscomb BV: Inspiring right attitudes in COPD outpatients (an interview), Respir Ther 2(3):2-3, 7, 1976.

Gray FD et al: Planning practical therapy for your COPD patient, Patient Care 8(4):104-135, 1974.

Gray FD et al: Educating your COPD patient in proper care, Patient Care 8(4):136-144, 1974.

Hopp J and Gerken C: Making an educational diagnosis to improve patient education, Respir Care (28)11:1456, Nov 1983.

Lazes PM: Health education project guides outpatients to active self-care, Hospitals: JAHA 51:81-86, Feb 1977.

Mclean DL et al: Self administration of medical modalities (SAMM): another method of rehabilitation education, Respir Care 28(11):1462, Nov 1983.

Moser K et al: Shortness of breath: a guide to better living and breathing, ed 3, St Louis, 1983, The CV Mosby Co.

Pennsylvania Society for Respiratory Therapy Inc: Respiratory home care procedure manual, Hershey, Pa, 1983, The Society.

Ransom J: Pulmonary home care . . . Your guide to more comfortable breathing, Kansas City, Mo, 1980, Baptist Memorial Hospital.

Seiler LH: The COPD patient's quality of life: can it be improved by patient education? Study conducted for the American Lung Association, 1-24, 58-66, 1979, The Association.

Steckel SB and Swain MA: Contracting with patients to improve compliance, Hospitals: JAHA 51:81-84, 1977.

CHAPTER 4

Ventilation retraining and relaxation in pulmonary disorders

VENTILATION

Ventilation, the movement of air into and out of the lungs, is caused by the contraction and relaxation of the diaphragm. As the diaphragm contracts, the superior-inferior aspect of the chest increases, and the contents of the upper abdomen are pushed outward. At this same time, the lower ribs expand increasing the anterior-posterior aspect of the chest. During quiet breathing this is all the movement necessary to ventilate normal lungs adequately and maintain homeostasis. When ventilatory requirements increase, other muscles add to alveolar ventilation.

The diaphragm is the most efficient muscle in the ventilation process. Its contraction provides adequate alveolar ventilation with a minimum of energy expenditure. The box on p. 53 lists the sequence of events during normal quiet breathing. Table 4-1 lists the muscles involved in quiet breathing and the additional muscles needed during times of increased demand for ventilation. During quiet breathing the external intercostal muscles can contribute to inspiration. During exhalation, usually a passive activity, the internal intercostal muscles may be involved. As energy requirements increase, all of the ventilatory muscles become active. The diaphragm, external intercostals, and accessory muscles, such as the sternocleidomastoid, trapezius, scalenes, and pectoralis major, contribute to inspiratory volume. When ventilatory demand increases, exhalation is no longer passive but involves the abdominal muscles such as the rectus abdominis, transversus abdominis, and internal and external obliques. The internal intercostals also help to expel air from the lungs. Proper function of these ventilatory muscles ensures adequate alveolar ventilation during a variety of circumstances.

During a normal day a person moves approximately 8640 liters of air into and out of the lungs, ~2052 gallons (12 breaths/min × 0.5 L/breath = 6 L/min × 1440 min/day = 8640 L/day/~3.8 L/gal = 2052 gal/day). O_2, which makes up 21% of inhaled air, enters the blood, is transported to working muscles and organs, and ultimately is used during metabolism. CO_2 is added to exhaled air from the blood returning from the body's cells. The amount of O_2 that is taken into all of the body's cells over a period of time is a measure of the body's energy requirements at that time. Approximately

---

SEQUENCE OF EVENTS DURING NORMAL, AT-REST INSPIRATION

1. The diaphragm contracts, pushing the contents of upper abdomen outward.
2. The diaphragm moves the ribs up and out on each side of the chest.
3. The upper chest rises slightly.

Table 4-1 Muscle involvement during quiet ventilation and increased ventilatory demand

	Inspiration	Expiration
Normal ventilation	Diaphragm External intercostals	Passive Relaxation of contracted muscles Occasional use of internal intercostals
Breathing at increased rates and depths of ventilation	Diaphragm External intercostals Accessory muscles (sterno-cleidomastoid, trapezius, scalenes, pectoralis major)	Abdominal muscles (rectus abdominis, transversus abdominis, internal and external oblique) Internal intercostals

360 L of oxygen is used per day by a normal person performing daily activities (0.25 L/min $\times$ 1440 min/day). A person must inhale 8640 L of air to provide the body with the required 360 L of O_2. This means that 24 L of air must be inhaled for each liter of O_2 consumed. The person with COPD must move a much greater number of liters of air into and out of the lungs to obtain the same level of oxygen consumption (Vo_2).

EFFICIENCY OF VENTILATION

A term used to describe the relationship between ventilation and oxygen consumption is *ventilatory equivalent*. This value can be expressed for O_2 consumed or CO_2 produced, Vo_{2eq} and Vco_{2eq}, respectively. (Vo_{2eq} can help to predict achievable energy expenditure and to develop an exercise prescription. [See Chapter 5.]) Generally the ventilatory equivalent, an indication of ventilatory efficiency, is the amount of ventilation required for a given level of energy expended. The lower the amount of air that must move through the lungs for each liter of oxygen consumed, the more efficient the ventilatory mechanism. A normal resting ventilatory equivalent for O_2 is 20 to 25 L of air per liter of oxygen consumed. (See the box on p. 54.) The relationship of ventilation to metabolism is fairly constant during a wide range of normal activities. During extreme exertion, such as running a race, the ventilatory equivalent increases even in a normal person as the ventilatory mechanism begins to approach its limits. A patient with COPD may have a ventilatory equivalent for O_2 as high as 30 to 50 L of air per

---
SAMPLE CALCULATION OF VENTILATORY EQUIVALENT _____

Given: 6.0 L of air/min and 0.25 L V_{O_2}/min

Ventilatory equivalent: $\dfrac{6.0}{0.25}$ = 24 L/L

---

liter of oxygen consumed, depending on the severity of that patient's ventilatory limitation.

The ventilatory equivalent expresses the relationship between the mechanism for ventilation, the lung-thorax bellows, and the level of metabolism or energy requirements in the body, and V_{O_2}. It is an expression of the *efficiency* of ventilation. As the system becomes less efficient, the ratio increases and more work must be done in breathing to achieve a similar level of V_{O_2}. Increased patient compliance and the loss of elasticity in the lungs of the patient with emphysema contribute to elevated ventilatory equivalent and loss of efficiency.

An elevated ventilatory equivalent in a pulmonary disorder requires one of two adjustments by the patient: ventilation can be increased to maintain the same O_2 intake required for activity, or the V_{O_2} requirements can be reduced by stopping the activity or slowing the activity level. It is apparent that the first option increases the work of breathing and the second option means a change in lifestyle.

VENTILATION RETRAINING FOR THE PATIENT WITH COPD

Dyspnea and the elevated work of breathing (WOB) that a patient with an obstructive pulmonary disorder experiences can be appreciated better by people without the disorder if they perform a simple experiment: walk up several flights of stairs while wearing a nose clip and inhaling and exhaling through a straw in your mouth. The increased difficulty of breathing through the straw will mimic the breathing resistance experienced by a patient with COPD. Now fill your lungs completely with air until you feel a stretching sensation in your chest, then exhale only a small amount of air, less than 1 L. Maintain a normal tidal ventilation, approximately 500 ml, at this point in vital capacity for as long as possible. Shortly after beginning this maneuver, fatigue from increased WOB will be experienced. It is uncomfortable when compared with normal tidal ventilation at a functional residual capacity (FRC). The increased residual volume of patients with COPD forces them to breathe at levels higher than normal because of air trapping.

The patient with COPD accommodates the increased work of breathing by making small changes in breathing over a period of years. This adaptation, or accommodation, has physiologic, social, and psychologic consequences. Health-care practitioners must be aware of these accommodations to deal effectively with the patient's problems and to rehabilitate the patient. The patient will need to learn to breathe in a different manner, to control breathing, and to coordinate breathing with all the ADL.

The primary goal in ventilation retraining is to enable the person with the pulmonary disorder to learn to control breathing in a variety of situations. Mastering controlled breathing requires both practice and reinforcement of appropriate breathing patterns. Controlled breathing requires the individual to attain a pattern of breathing that is paced according to the activity being performed and thus minimizes energy use for ventilation. Ultimately this improved breathing efficiency translates into better tolerance of activities. This is not a simple task and will require time, diligent practice, and follow-up.

During breathing practice sessions, emphasis should be on the breathing patterns that mimic those used during ADL. Particular attention should be paid to ventilation during upper-body motion or activities that involve lifting, reaching, pulling, pushing, and personal-hygiene activities such as brushing hair, bathing, shaving, and bowel movements.

Two components make up the foundation of ventilation retraining in COPD. The first component is the use of pursed-lip breathing and diaphragmatic/abdominal breathing. These techniques of breathing may sound easy to do and explain, but they are difficult for the patient to learn and perform, especially when experiencing dyspnea. The second aspect of breathing to be included in ventilation training is coordinating breathing with body movements during activities and recognizing limits to breathing control. A patient's practice, motivation, and diligence in learning the technique and encouragement from the people coaching him are essential to the mastery of the fundamentals of ventilation retraining. The benefits to a patient of these methods of ventilation are listed below:

1. Decrease respiratory rate (RR)
2. Decrease Pa_{CO_2}
3. Increase alveolar ventilation
4. Improve ventilatory equivalent

Pursed-lip breathing

Many patients with an obstructive lung disorder have discovered by themselves that if they offer a slight resistance to exhalation with the lips, the sensation of SOB can be reduced. The goals of pursed-lip breathing are listed in the box on p. 56. The reasons for the effectiveness of pursed-lip breathing are not completely clear, but it is helpful to appreciate what it is that contributes to the early collapse of airways and subsequent air trapping.

The loss of lung elasticity in COPD and aging, along with bronchial muscle constriction and edema, all contribute to the earlier-than-normal closure of small distal

_____ **GOALS OF PURSED-LIP BREATHING** _____

Slow respiratory rate (RR)

Prolong exhalation (I:E > 1:2)

Allow "more complete" emptying (decreased FRC) and refilling of the distal airways in the lungs

Provide a mechanism for the patient to control respiratory efforts during periods of dyspnea

airways. Tissue pressures in the lung that surround the airways (intrathoracic pressure) during exhalation can exceed the pressure inside the airways themselves. When this happens, the airways collapse, preventing movement of gas out of those lung units distal to the obstruction. Pursed-lip breathing seems to generate resistance to airflow at the mouth that is transmitted as pressure into the airways. This allows for a slightly positive pressure, relative to the surrounding tissue pressures, inside the airways during exhalation. The airways will still collapse, but the collapse will occur at a later time in the expiratory phase. More air will have been exhaled and subsequently a larger volume of air can be inhaled into these lung units than otherwise would have been possible. The relative positive pressure present inside the airways of the lungs has been expressed as a movement of the "equal-pressure point" into the airways from its normal position at the lips. The result of breathing with pursed lips during exhalation in the person with early airway collapse is a decrease in his FRC and an ability to increase alveolar minute ventilation.

The amount of time a patient spends exhaling should be more than twice the amount of time spent inhaling (I:E ratio > 1:2), and a respiratory rate (RR) of < 20 breaths/min should be maintained. These ventilation traits contribute to a decrease in the amount of air trapped in the distal lung units. Pursed-lip breathing can help a patient to maintain an expiratory time and RR at this level. The overall effect of the slower RR and appropriate I:E ratio is a decrease in the WOB, less fatigue, decreased episodes of dyspnea, and a feeling of increased relaxation and control for the patient.

Training in pursed-lip breathing

The emphasis of training in pursed-lip breathing should be relaxed exhalation. The technique is best learned when the patient is at rest and is experiencing no distress. The patient should discontinue trying to learn these methods if distracted by them while in the early stages of learning to control breathing with activity. Inspired breaths should be near a normal tidal breath. The tendency of many patients is to inhale more deeply than normal. The patient should breathe through the nose, using the diaphragm; exhalation should be as passive as possible, through the mouth with the lips pursed. Air should come out of the lungs more slowly because the lips are pursed. The patient should make no effort to prolong exhalation by holding breath in the lungs and letting it out slowly.

To help the patient recognize his breathing pattern, rate, and rhythm, have him inhale through the nose and exhale through the mouth without resistance for a minute of normal breathing. Next, have him begin to resist exhalation slightly, using the lips. He should feel a sensation in the lips but not in other parts of the upper airway, such as the cheeks. The patient should strive to maintain this resistance throughout the entire time he is exhaling, even if he may not "feel" air coming out, for example, near the end of exhalation. The most frequent error in pursed-lip breathing is premature relaxation of the lips and subsequent loss of resistance near the end of exhalation. Early relaxation of the lips can undermine the benefit of pursed-lip breathing. Airway collapse occurs at low lung volumes, especially the low volumes in the lungs at the end of exhalation. When resistance is lost prematurely at the end of exhalation, some of the air that would have been exhaled is trapped in the airways. The patient can provide resistance at the lips by puckering them or by stretching them tightly across the mouth. The less conspicuous the patient feels when performing the technique, the greater the likelihood he will use it in public when necessary.

There are some important points to watch for when training a person in pursed-lip breathing. The patient must realize that it will be necessary to perform the technique for several minutes when in distress before experiencing relief. During the attempt to gain control of breathing using pursed lips during exhalation, the patient must observe several rules of pursed-lip breathing: (1) The patient should not "blow out" or allow the cheeks to expand when exhaling. (2) The narrowing, or pursing, of the lips must be maintained for the duration of exhalation. (3) The patient should exhale in a manner as passive as possible under the circumstances (Fig. 4-1).

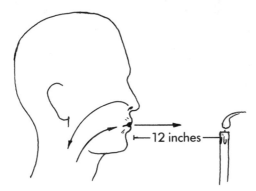

Fig. 4-1 The patient should practice pursed-lip breathing without "blowing" by exhaling through pursed lips toward a candle placed about 12 in from the mouth. The flame should only bend; it should not be extinguished by exhalation.

A whistling sound produced during exhalation is often an indication that the patient is not exhaling in a passive manner. The force generated by blowing increases the transpulmonary pressure, which contributes to the collapse of airways. The expiratory flow rate from a patient with COPD may be below 100 ml/min at the end of exhalation. The resistance to exhalation offered at these low flow rates does not produce the same obvious sensation in the lips as is experienced at the higher flow rates earlier in exhalation. Many patients stop resisting exhalation at this point by relaxing the pursed lips. The effect of resistance to exhalation is lost before the lungs can be emptied sufficiently. Initially the patient may feel that passive exhalation during an episode of SOB is impossible to achieve. But practice and training help the patient to realize that passive exhalation through pursed lips is possible and that such control of breathing is worth the effort and time required to learn it.

Inhalation and exhalation should be timed according to the patient's own cadence for breathing. This counting of inspiratory time and expiratory time should be consistent, rhythmic, and even. At times the patient may tend to count more quickly for exhalation than for inhalation. This difference will not achieve the desired result of an exhalation time that is 2 times the count of inspiration and a RR that is less than 20 breaths/min. While at rest and comfortably positioned the patient can, with practice, achieve a slow rate of respiration and a prolonged exhalation time. A RR of 10 to 12 breaths/min and an I:E ratio of 1:5 are possible goals. The patient should not be forced to adhere to the counting rhythm of the health-care provider training him. If the patient has difficulty achieving a smooth, rhythmic count, a metronome may be helpful in establishing a rhythm for the counting.

Once this breathing pattern and rhythm have been mastered, the patient can begin to incorporate them into activities and exercises. During physical activity an increase in RR is probably necessary to accommodate the increased demand for O_2 and elimination of CO_2. At some point the increased RR may require that the patient inhale through the mouth instead of through the nose. The fundamentals of controlled breathing, an exhalation time more than 2 times that of inhalation and a respiratory rate of less than 20 breaths/min, should always be observed. If either of these elements cannot be maintained, the patient should slow or stop the activity while continuing to practice pursed-lip breathing until he is again in control (see the box on p. 59).

Diaphragmatic breathing

Diaphragmatic breathing is generally incorporated into retraining in breathing patterns and often accompanies pursed-lip breathing. Following are goals of diaphragmatic breathing:

Improved ventilation (lower $Paco_2$, possibly increased Pao_2)

Prevention of atelectasis

Decreased WOB

Increased cough effectiveness

Assistance in patient relaxation

############### IMPORTANT POINTS ABOUT PURSED-LIP BREATHING ###############

1. Do not *blow* air out during exhalation.
   Blowing air out increases pressure around airways and contributes to further air trapping.
2. Coordinate breathing with activities.
   Pace breathing with the activity according to its demands and rhythm. Exhalation should never be $<2 \times$ inspiration, and a RR of <20 breaths/min should be maintained.
3. Always exhale upon any exertion.
   Avoid performing Valsalva's maneuver when lifting, reaching, pulling, or pushing. Do not hold breath and strain.

The reduced energy expenditure and slower RR resulting from the use of the diaphragm can be very relaxing. Some patients may have a difficult time in coordinating both pursed-lip and diaphragmatic breathing, and in this situation the emphasis should be placed on using pursed lips, prolonging exhalation, and slowing RR.

In many pulmonary disorders the diaphragm of the patient has a flattened shape as opposed to the normal domed shape. This shape contributes to the diaphragm's ventilatory inefficiency. The flattened diaphragm has lost some of its mechanical advantage for increasing the anterior-posterior and superior-inferior movement of the thorax. Throughout the many years the pulmonary disorder was developing, use of the accessory muscles of the upper chest, neck, abdomen, and back has become routine for the COPD patient. For these muscles to maintain adequate ventilation, they must work at a faster RR with lower volumes. This often causes these accessory muscles to become larger and less efficient by themselves for ventilation. Accessory muscles fatigue easily, contributing to dyspnea and respiratory failure. If the diaphragm can be used as the primary means of ventilation, increased ventilation required during activities can be provided by the accessory muscles.

It is not clear whether actual improvement in diaphragmatic function can be accomplished through diaphragmatic-breathing training alone. What may actually occur is training and strengthening of the abdominal muscles to move the diaphragm. The diaphragm is moved by the displacement of the abdominal contents, which pulls or pushes the diaphragm into or away from the thorax, thereby ventilating the lungs. The sniff test or percussion of the posterior chest during deep inhalation and exhalation can allow the health-care provider to assess diaphragmatic movement. An abdominal breathing pattern may improve diaphragmatic function, eliminate the inefficient upper-chest breathing pattern, and contribute to improved ventilation.

Training in diaphragmatic breathing

Training a patient to use the diaphragm more fully when breathing is not as easy as it may first appear. The technique and the training procedure should be explained to

---

POSITIONS FOR PRACTICING DIAPHRAGMATIC BREATHING

Practice 3 times each day for 10 minutes each time in a quiet, nondistracting environment.

Easiest positions

Lying down with or without weights on abdomen
Sitting in straight-backed chair
Standing with good posture

Hardest positions

Walking slowly or with a normal gait
Stair climbing (pause as needed)
Exercising

---

the patient's satisfaction. Diligent practice is required to make diaphragmatic and pursed-lip breathing habitual breathing patterns.

For this breathing pattern to become habitual, the patient must follow a routine for practicing each skill. A regular time of day and amount of time should be set aside for practicing diaphragmatic and pursed-lip breathing while lying down, sitting, standing, and walking. Although the patient may be able to perform these techniques lying down and in other resting positions, it will be a challenge to breathe in this manner while sitting, standing, or walking (see the box on p. 60).

Good posture can be an aid to better breathing. Standing and sitting erect allows gravity to assist the movement of the diaphragm and abdominal contents during inhalation. Initially the semi-Fowler's or Fowler's position (supine, head elevated 20° to 45°, knees bent and supported by pillows) is a comfortable and relaxing position.

The suggestions for patient education given in Chapter 3 should be used for training and educating the patient in these breathing patterns. The health-care practitioner should demonstrate the breathing pattern for several minutes to the patient and his family. Next, the patient should try the procedure while the practitioner "coaches" him. The practitioner should demonstrate again, and the patient should try the procedure a second time, again with "coaching." Once the patient appears to have grasped the concept, even though he may not perform each procedure perfectly, the practitioner should prescribe several practice sessions each day. The practitioner should encourage the patient to perform this type of breathing throughout the day but always to set aside a certain time to concentrate on it during the prescribed practice sessions.

Hands-on and verbal coaching can be helpful when the patient is trying to learn to use the diaphragm more effectively for breathing. The patient must first learn where the diaphragm is located. The health-care practitioner can help in finding its location by placing her hands on the patient's hands while the patient's hands are on the lateral

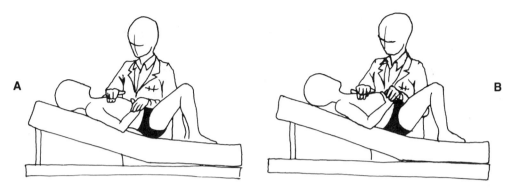

Fig. 4-2 Hand placement for training in diaphragmatic breathing. The patient should place one hand on the chest and the other hand on the upper abdomen, below the xiphoid process and just touching the lower ribs. The practitioner's hands should be placed on top of the patient's. **A,** The practitioner should gently depress the upper abdomen during exhalation, especially at the end of exhalation. At the end of exhalation and just before the beginning of inhalation, the practitioner should release the pressure of the hand quickly and allow the lower ribs to "spring" out when the patient inhales. **B,** The practitioner should not remove the hand completely from its position on the patient but should release the downward pressure.

aspect of his upper abdomen. The lowest ribs should be felt under the patient's hands. The patient should then use his nose to "sniff." The quick, outward motion of the lower ribs is the diaphragm contracting. This action should be repeated until the patient is certain that he can locate the diaphragm.

During coaching sessions in diaphragmatic breathing, the patient places one hand on the chest and the other on the upper abdomen, below the xyphoid process and just touching the lower ribs. The practitioner places her hands on top of the patient's hands (Fig. 4-2). Ask him to relax and breathe normally for a minute or two and to "feel" how he is breathing, establishing a rate and rhythm. The health-care provider follows the patient's breathing pattern for several minutes and explains to the patient that she will intervene with the patient's breathing by placing gentle pressure on the upper abdomen during exhalation. This pressure may further assist the patient to become conscious of the motion of his diaphragm and abdomen and his breathing rhythm. Continue to press gently on the upper abdomen during exhalation, especially at the end of exhalation. At the end of exhalation and just before the beginning of inhalation, the health-care provider releases the pressure of her hand quickly and allows the abdomen and lower ribs to "spring" out when the patient inhales. She does not remove her hand completely from its position on the patient, but reduces the downward pressure. This procedure is repeated several times, and the health-care provider encourages the patient to "breathe into her hand," to feel the pushing of his abdomen out with the diaphragm and sensation of inhalation. Repeat this procedure with each breath for several minutes, slowing RR.

PROBLEMS TO AVOID
IN PURSED-LIP AND DIAPHRAGMATIC BREATHING

Avoid forced exhalation; it should be slow, relaxed, and passive.
Do not artificially prolong exhalation by letting air out slowly.
Slow RR to about 10/min at rest to avoid hyperventilation (indicated by dizziness and
tingling fingers).
Do not arch the back to push out the abdomen.
Do not use chest muscles for normal inhalation.

The patient may need a period of rest from the concentrated effort. If the diaphragmatic pattern of breathing is lost, stop, relax, and then begin again. The focus of the patient's attention during breathing should be the sensation of diaphragmatic and upper abdominal movement during inhalation and the reduction of chest motion. When breathing is done properly, the patient often will sense a dramatic reduction in chest motion and be surprised that he is adequately ventilated with such little effort and abdominal motion. Although it is best to inhale through the nose and exhale through the mouth with lips pursed during this breathing technique, it may be necessary to hold some of this coordination until later training sessions. Prescribed and coached training sessions initially can be short (approximately 5 to 10 min) because it may be difficult to maintain the breathing pattern for longer periods. Weights, 1 to 2 kg initially, may be used on the upper abdomen to allow the patient to work against a resistance to sense abdominal movement. This resistive work can eventually be a means of strength training for the abdominal muscles and perhaps the diaphragm. The added weights to provide resistance against which to work the upper abdomen and diaphragm are similar in function to the hand of the health-care provider and can be helpful during training while at home.

As the patient masters the diaphragmatic breathing pattern in one position, he should progress to greater difficulty levels (Table 4-1). Each position can be practiced for 2 to 3 min of the practice session. The goal of this training is to allow this pattern of breathing to be performed all day in a variety of circumstances. The health-care provider should watch for problems such as those listed in the box above during training in diaphragmatic and pursed-lip breathing. If the patient complains of an increase in SOB or fatigue, this may indicate that he is performing the technique incorrectly and perhaps training should be repeated. As always, encouragement and positive reinforcement are important during training.

CONTROL OF BREATHING AND PACING WITH ADL

The overall goal for breathing retraining is to allow the patient to have a slowed, relaxed, and efficient manner of breathing that can be integrated into numerous ADL.

The patient should practice pursed-lip and diaphragmatic/abdominal breathing while walking in a crowd, alone on level surfaces, and up hills or stairs. It may be necessary to include gait training with training in the use of these breathing techniques. This integration of training allows the patient to pace his walking and use the cadence of his walking as a mechanism for counting inhalation and exhalation time. For example, the patient should inhale for two steps and exhale for four steps, for an I:E ratio of 1:2. When the patient becomes fatigued or short of breath or finds he must breathe at a RR > 20 breaths/min during activities, he should slow down or stop and continue pursed-lip and diaphragmatic breathing to regain breathing control.

Often a patient will discover for himself how to coordinate breathing with various activities. Activities that involve upper-body or arm motion are usually the most difficult to coordinate with breathing. As mentioned earlier, the patient should exhale through pursed lips when lifting, reaching, or pulling or pushing an object. Activities such as lifting a bag of groceries, reaching for a can high on a kitchen shelf, pushing a lawnmower or a broom, or pulling up the covers on a bed should be performed while exhaling through pursed lips. These types of motions should be practiced. After any exertion, a momentary pause to inhale and exhale, a "rest breath," should be taken before continuing activity.

Coordination of breathing with activities of personal hygiene, such as showers, bowel movements, and shaving requires practice and patience. The patient should be encouraged to discuss household chores and other activities with which he is trying to coordinate breathing. Discussion of these activities allows the patient and staff to devise a means of controlling breathing or altering the activity. In general, by taking a little extra time when performing household activities and keeping in mind the basic principles of breathing techniques, the patient can train himself to coordinate and control breathing during activities.

VENTILATION RETRAINING EXERCISES

During early training sessions exercises should be simple and should require little energy expenditure. The focus of these sessions should be mastering the control (pacing) and coordination of breathing with the motion involved in the activity. This control includes using the diaphragm, minimizing chest motion during inspiration, and exhaling in a relaxed, passive manner through pursed lips. Breathing can be paced rhythmically with the cadence and motion of many exercises or activities. The primary objective of any ventilation retraining exercise (VRE) is not to increase the strength of the ventilatory muscles but to develop control over ventilation during activities. This may require a patient to unlearn one means of breathing and replace it with a more efficient and effective breathing pattern. (See pursed-lip and diaphragmatic breathing, beginning on p. 55.)

Calisthenic exercises can be modified to decrease the energy required to perform them and then used as a ventilation retraining exercise. Several of these exercises are

SUGGESTED EXERCISES FOR VENTILATION RETRAINING	
Shoulder shrugs	Scissor kick
Arm circles	Sit-ups
Forward bends	Shoulder raises
Head circles	Side bends
Arm swinging	Reaching and rotation

given in the box on p. 64, and more are illustrated in Appendix G. For example, such a reduction can be achieved by going slowly through the motions, sitting down during the exercise, or keeping arms down as opposed to including them in the exercise. By reducing the amount of energy required to perform an exercise, the patient is able to concentrate on the control and coordination of breathing with the motion of the body rather than on the work of the muscles involved. After a number of practice sessions, when the patient has mastered coordination of breathing with exercise, it may be possible to increase the intensity of the exercise to achieve an exercise goal. The patient may already know how to perform the motions in the calisthenic exercise, so practice sessions should focus on controlling breathing during the activity. The exercise tables in Appendix G are provided as suggestions for calisthenic exercises that have been modified to be used as ventilation retraining activities. The health-care staff and the patient will need to use some creativity when adapting the exercises to achieve the goal of retraining the patient in breathing patterns and activity. As a general rule, simplifying the motions, reducing arm and shoulder movement, and having the patient sit or lie down will provide a good beginning point for performing calisthenic exercises as VREs.

It is recommended for planning ventilation retraining that the patient allow at least 20 to 30 min every day for performing a variety of VREs. Variety in the exercises is important in maintaining the patient's interest and motivation. The patient may become bored with the exercises or consider them so routine that little thought of his breathing is required. The patient should be encouraged to think of exercises that he would like to do. Appropriate modifications should be suggested if necessary, and the patient's input about how to perform the VRE should be considered. Having input into the ventilation-retraining aspect of his rehabilitation program gives the patient some control over program activities. When putting together a rehabilitation program, the staff should remember that the patient and his family are being trained in program activities so that they can provide care at home.

The activities and exercises in ventilation retraining should mimic as much as possible the activities and exercises performed in everyday life, such as lifting, reaching, pulling, and pushing. For example, if the patient has a shelf in the kitchen that he frequently accesses for supplies or utensils, exercises that incorporate lifting and reaching will help him to perform this activity. Once the patient and family have been interviewed, tasks that are troublesome for the patient can be identified. Perhaps there is a task that the patient would like to be able to perform but avoids because of his breathing problem. Obtaining this kind of information facilitates individualization of program exercises. It also provides a short-term, measurable goal for the patient. This goal can be helpful in motivating the patient and monitoring progress in ventilation retraining and other program activities.

The idea that a patient will need to learn a dozen or more modified calisthenic exercises, master breathing control during the motions required in the exercises, and then use these same exercises at a later time to increase his strength and coordination may be difficult for a patient to accept. The patient with a pulmonary disability and breathing limitation cannot train and exercise at the same level at which people without these problems would. Breathing control must first be mastered and then built upon. Practical application of breathing control in everyday situations is the emphasis of the activities used for ventilation retraining. When exercises in a ventilation-retraining session are designed, the patient's desires and interests should be considered. The ultimate goal is that the patient will begin to train himself, with guidance from the members of the rehabilitation and health-care teams.

Coaching, especially during the early sessions of ventilation retraining, builds the patient's confidence in his ability to control his breathing. The importance of thorough ventilation retraining in the rehabilitation of pulmonary patients cannot be over-emphasized. Breathing control, improved breathing efficiency, and adaptation to ADL are the foundation for the long-term benefits of pulmonary rehabilitation.

PURPOSE OF RELAXATION TRAINING IN COPD

A major goal for a patient with COPD is to achieve and maintain a reduction in anxiety and apprehension, which can contribute to SOB just as physical exertion or psychosocial stress does. Stress is a part of life and can be harmful or helpful, depending on the circumstances and how the patient reacts to it. Problems with stress arise when its intensity goes beyond the patient's ability to cope with it. Many patients benefit from mastery of a relaxation technique to use during stressful situations. The benefits of relaxation are most apparent during an anxiety-producing situation. But for the patient to experience the benefits of relaxation, he must learn the skill and practice it during periods of relative calm.

Tension (stress or apprehension) can be high in intensity yet short in duration, as in a pleasant or unpleasant surprise. A situation, such as exercise or a social engagement, may require the expenditure of a short burst of energy. Although this type of stress must be considered when training for relaxation, long-term stress, such as the stress brought on by a chronic disability or disease, marital discord, or social isolation and loneliness, should be the major consideration when training a patient in relaxation.

Frequent occurrence of short-term stressors that stimulate the body's fight-or-flight mechanism can lead to ulcers, headaches, somatic pain, skin rashes, bronchospasm, and heart palpitations. Long-term occurrence of stressors tends to reduce the body's defense mechanisms, thus lowering resistance to infection. Stress also impairs the body's ability to adapt to changes in the environment. Patients with chronic lung disease or those who find themselves under continuous stress often complain of exhaustion and low energy levels.

One relaxation technique may be useful in a variety of situations and types of stress. The patient may prefer one technique over another and it will take a good amount of time for anyone to learn several techniques. Selection of the first techniques learned is important, but the patient should be open to other methods of relaxation.

Patients who master relaxation training tend to have a greater sense of control over their symptoms and their life situation. The patient is able to develop better coping mechanisms for dealing with physical and psychosocial stressors. A relaxed patient is better able to focus on the tasks set before him, thereby improving concentration and learning the skills needed in rehabilitation and self-care.

General relaxation and relaxation of specific muscle groups reduce oxygen consumption, decrease blood pressure, and foster a sense of well-being in the patient. Through discussions with the patient and his family, anxiety-producing situations can be identified, and suggestions can be developed to deal with each situation.

Training in relaxation techniques allows the patient to focus on something other than the anxiety-producing situation. This shift in attention often reduces the importance of the stressor and allows the patient to concentrate on maintaining control.

A limited amount of stress is a necessary part of functioning in today's society. Few patients can relax fully at will, and it may be very difficult for a patient to identify a state of relaxation. Each patient should attempt to identify levels of stress that are enough to maintain function in society but not too much to cope with. This is difficult, but an experienced health-care provider can provide valuable assistance to the patient, especially through open discussions, in determining these levels.

The patient needs to be taught to recognize stress and its effects. Stress may show as jitteriness, SOB, muscle tension in the shoulders and neck, and headaches. Other signs of stress are insomnia, depression, and a lack of interest in activities. The family and other people who have contact with the patient should be observant for signs of high levels of stress, such as high alcohol intake every day and throughout the day, eating excessively or not at all, complaints of diarrhea or constipation, restlessness, or lethargy.

Although a high level of independent action on the part of the patient undergoing rehabilitation is desirable, this increase in decision-making may be a stressor in itself. The patient should not be allowed to focus on himself and his own situation for too long. It is important that the patient have a support network of friends, family, health-care workers, and social workers to bring into the decision-making process. A routine of daily care and stability in the home environment can provide a base for dealing with stressors generated by the "outside world" or by the disorder. The patient may need assistance in identifying specific approaches to stressful situations. Several suggestions should be made to the patient in general terms, and more specific suggestions should be made through discussions and interviews with the patient.

FOUR BASIC REQUIREMENTS FOR DEVELOPMENT OF RELAXATION SKILLS

An environment in which a patient can practice and learn relaxation techniques is important. Generally the best locations are free from interruptions, out of harsh light, quiet, and familiar to the patient. Many different techniques can be used to encourage relaxation, but four common conditions have been identified that assist the patient's relaxation during any of the stress-reduction techniques.

1. *A quiet, calm environment.* The location used for training should be as free of distractions as possible. It should be one in which the patient is comfortable and familiar with the surroundings. Subdued lighting (not *too* dark) may be helpful.
2. *A mental focal point.* A word, phrase, or thought can be a mental focal point for relaxation. Gazing at a particular object or spot on a wall can also help the patient to concentrate on a focal point. The patient may also focus on the rhythmic movement or sound of breathing. During periods of relaxation, most people's minds tend to wander. A patient learning relaxation techniques should not fight this natural wandering. He should allow the extraneous thoughts to drift through his mind and return to his focal point upon realizing he has wandered.
3. *A passive attitude.* If the patient worries about how well he is relaxing, relaxation will never be achieved. It is important that the patient understand that mastering these techniques takes time. Each patient will have distracting, extraneous thoughts, which should be allowed simply to drift through the mind as the patient attempts to return to the focal point. Time and a proper mental attitude are more important than effort and concentration.
4. *A comfortable position.* The patient should be in a familiar position that reduces muscular effort as much as possible. Sitting, lying, or reclining in a chair are all acceptable positions. The patient should avoid the tendency to fall asleep during relaxation sessions. It is important for the patient to know what it "feels like" to be relaxed so that this sensation can be reproduced in stressful situations.

PROGRESSIVE MUSCLE RELAXATION

Progressive relaxation exercises are a common method of promoting relaxation. This technique involves the systematic contraction and relaxation of muscle groups. Muscles should be contracted to a maximum level and for a short period of time, approximately 3 to 5 seconds. The relaxation that follows the maximal contraction

_____ **GENERAL SUGGESTIONS FOR RELAXATION TRAINING** _____

1. Avoid stress-producing situations.
   If stressors, such as crowds, heavy traffic, or a living situation, cannot be avoided, the following suggestions may be helpful:
   A change in the patient's attitude toward the home environment or the stressors may be necessary. The most appropriate attitude is acceptance of stressors that cannot be changed and recognition of those that can be changed.
   Break a situation into components that can be controlled by the patient and those that cannot be controlled. Plan for the management of the controllable aspects.
2. Exercise regularly.
   Regular exercise is important in relieving tension, but it can increase tension if done improperly. The patient should never push herself beyond clearly identified physical limits.
   Rhythmic, repetitive motion such as walking at a constant speed, pedaling a stationary bicycle at a constant speed and resistance, and performing basic calisthenic exercises can be helpful.
3. Set aside time regularly to relax.
   Lie down quietly in a semidark room with no interruptions for 20 or 30 min daily.
   Though sleeping is not the same as relaxing, some patients take a nap to reduce anxiety levels.
   If the patient requires O_2 during activities, it should also be administered during relaxation sessions and sleep periods.
   Perform relaxation-training techniques regularly, especially during stressful situations.
4. Develop outside interests.
   Evaluate talents, abilities, or interests the patient has.
   Enjoyable activities help to shift the patient's focus of attention from himself and his stressors toward other people and activities. Generally a hobby should be different from other activities performed on a routine basis, such as work.
   Many older patients have developed over time skills and talents they can share with others. Placing the COPD patient in a role in which he is teaching others something that they enjoy can be very beneficial.

should be as complete as possible and last 3 to 4 times longer than contraction. The following areas of the body are frequently targeted during this method of progressive relaxation:

Face and head
Neck
Shoulders
Upper arms
Chest and upper back
Hands and forearms
Abdomen and lower back

Thighs and buttocks

Calves and ankles

Feet and toes

The patient may progress in contracting the muscles from the head to the feet or from the feet to the head. If the patient experiences the greatest tension in the upper portion of the body, such as the neck and shoulders, progressive relaxation should begin at the head and work down. Particular emphasis should be placed on relaxing the muscles of the neck and shoulders because they are frequently used in breathing. These areas of the body often remain contracted as they become tense, decreasing their efficiency and increasing the need for O_2. Because the patient can become confused if too many specific muscle groups are identified, it is best to keep the initial discussion as simple as possible.

The patient should be able to feel the relaxation in each area as he progresses through the entire sequence. The sequence should be repeated until maximal relaxation of the whole body has been achieved or, in early phases of training, for about 20 to 30 min. Practice is essential for mastery of any relaxation technique. With time the patient will find it easier to perform each technique and will enjoy the benefits of relaxation more thoroughly. Initially relaxation training sessions should take place twice a day for 10 minutes each time. Once the basics of the technique have been learned, one 20-minute session each day may be sufficient to reinforce what has been learned and improve performance.

MENTAL IMAGERY IN RELAXATION

General body relaxation can also be achieved through the "painting" of a mental picture that is relaxing to the patient. Often a calm, soothing voice talking a patient through this mental process is helpful. Discover one of the patient's favorite places to relax, such as the mountains or the beach. The patient should then create for himself scenes and situations that are calming and stress-reducing. In general, warmth, pastoral scenery, and rhythmic noises, such as waves against the seashore or wind through the trees, help to create a relaxing mental image. The relaxation trainer should not require specific items for the patient's mental image but should encourage the patient to develop his own. Once the patient has created this image, he should enjoy it, noting how different areas of the body feel when relaxed. This relaxed sensation can then be drawn upon later during stressful situations. Tapes and records are available commercially for this type of relaxation training. Some of them include a soothing voice to lead the session; others simply supply background noise or music.

During a stressful situation in which breathing control is important, the patient can bring back this mental image to reduce anxiety. This technique can be particularly helpful in socially stressful situations, such as crowded elevators, long grocery-store lines, traffic jams, or parties. By dwelling on a calming mental picture, the patient can begin to experience relaxation and to control tension and breathing to some degree in a variety of situations.

OTHER RELAXATION TECHNIQUES

Many patients have found meditation to be helpful for promoting relaxation. Yoga exercise is another relaxation technique that has been found to be beneficial. Yoga's slow stretching and positioning while controlling breathing followed by relaxation from the position has been found to be a very pleasant and soothing experience. Many patients with lung disease who have practiced meditation or yoga have experienced relief of symptoms and better control of breathing.

Biofeedback can be used in relaxation training, especially to teach the patient to recognize a relaxed state. It is also helpful in achieving greater and greater depth of relaxation. Electromyography (EMG), galvanic skin response (GSR), and other biofeedback techniques, such as alpha waves, have been employed in relaxation training. These techniques can be very helpful, especially for patients who have difficulty recognizing that they are becoming relaxed. It is also possible through biofeedback to identify specific muscle groups for relaxation training. As mentioned earlier, the shoulder and neck muscles of the COPD patient are frequently in need of relaxation. By attaching electrodes to these muscle groups and monitoring their response during relaxation sessions, their function can be improved and recorded.

Slow, rhythmic exercise can also contribute to general relaxation of the body. But it is important to remember that fatigue is not relaxation. Modified calisthenic exercises, such as those listed in the box below and in Appendix H, that are performed in a rhythmic, repetitive fashion will stretch the muscle groups involved and promote relaxation.

Relaxation of specific muscle groups can improve breathing and somatic appearance and lower overall energy expenditure. The COPD patient should concentrate initially on relaxing specific muscle groups of the upper body, especially the shoulders,

---

MODIFIED RHYTHMIC EXERCISES FOR RELAXATION

Swinging the arms in large and small circles
Dangling the arms in front of the body and swinging them back and forth like a pendulum
"Drawing circles" in the air with the toes
Kicking lower legs outward while sitting on a high table or chair
Rotating the head
Shrugging shoulders
Rolling shoulders in large circles

neck, and back, to improve breathing. General relaxation allows the patient to develop coping mechanisms and a sense of control during anxiety-producing situations. A number of techniques are available to promote general body relaxation, but four conditions—a calm environment, a mental focal point, a passive attitude, and a comfortable position—are important for the success of any relaxation method.

BIBLIOGRAPHY

Anderson CL, Shankar PS, and Scott JH: Physiological significance of sternomastoid muscle contraction in chronic obstructive pulmonary disease, Respir Care 25(9):937-939, 1980.

Astrand P and Rodahl K: Textbook of work physiology, ed 2, New York, 1977, McGraw-Hill, Inc.

Bradley CA, Fleetham JA, and Anthonisen NR: Ventilatory control in patients with hypoxemia due to obstructive lung disease, Am Rev Respir Dis 120:21-30, 1979.

Casciari RJ et al: Effects of breathing retraining in patients with chronic obstructive pulmonary disease, Chest 79(4):393-398, 1981.

Davis MH et al: Relaxation training facilitated by biofeedback apparatus as a supplemental treatment in bronchial asthma, J Psychosom Res 17:121-128, 1973.

deVries HA et al: Efficacy of EMG biofeedback in relaxation training: a controlled study, Am J Phys Med 56(2):75-81, 1977.

Frownfelter DL: Breathing exercise and retraining, chest mobilization exercises, Chest physical therapy and pulmonary rehabilitation: an interdisciplinary approach 153-175, Chicago, 1978, Year Book Medical Publishers, Inc.

Hassett J: Teaching yourself to relax, Psychology Today, p 28, August 1978.

Hodgkin JE, Zorn E, and Connors G: Pulmonary rehabilitation: guidelines to success, Stoneham, Mass, 1984, Butterworth Publishers.

Motley HL: The effects of slow deep breathing on the blood gas exchange in emphysema, Am Rev Respir Dis 88:484-492, 1963.

Mueller RE, Petty TI, and Filley GF: Ventilation and arterial blood gas changes induced by pursed lips breathing, J Appl Physiol 28(6):784-789, 1970.

Pardy RL et al: Inspiratory muscle training compared with physiotherapy in patients with chronic airflow limitation, Am Rev Respir Dis 123:421-425, 1981.

Petty T et al: Intensive and rehabilitative respiratory care, ed 2, Philadelphia, 1974, Lea & Febiger.

Weiss RA and Karpovich PV: Energy cost of exercises for convalescents, Arch Phys Med 47:447-454, 1947.

CHAPTER 5

Exercise and reconditioning in pulmonary disorders

GENERAL CONCEPTS IN EXERCISE TRAINING

The relationship between the lungs, the heart and circulatory system, and the cells involved in metabolism is expressed in Fig. 5-1. These systems and exercising muscles are closely linked in metabolism. Each is important in the delivery of O_2 and nutrients (for energy) to the body's tissues and the removal of CO_2 and other waste products from the tissue as energy to perform work. A disorder affecting one system will affect the ability of the other systems to perform their functions.

O_2 is essential to proper cell function. The only way for oxygen to get into the body and exercising muscles and cells is through the lungs, which also act as the primary organ for removal of CO_2. Small amounts of CO_2 and other waste products of metabolism are removed from the body in other ways, such as in perspiration and urine.

Even if the concentration of O_2 in the atmosphere is adequate and the lungs are functioning correctly, the heart and circulatory system must also function correctly to ensure the delivery of oxygen to the tissues. The function of the heart as the blood pump and the blood vessels as the delivery pipeline can significantly affect the ability to exercise. Cardiovascular function is considered the primary exercise limitation in normal and trained individuals. Once the maximum cardiac output is attained, the patient will be unable to continue to achieve higher levels of energy expenditure. This is true whether the ventilatory (lung) or metabolic (muscle) work limit has been reached or not.

The muscles must be able to remove O_2 from the blood for metabolism and quickly deliver CO_2 and other waste products of metabolism to the blood for disposal. As the muscles contract, they squeeze the veins, thereby assisting in the return of CO_2-rich blood to the heart and lungs. The muscles doing the work need to have the proper types and numbers of muscle fibers and mitochondria and to be sufficiently vascularized to have the ability to perform the required work. The mechanical advantage and neuromuscular function (coordination) of work performance is also important.

Each of the body's systems plays a key role in exercise (work) performance. Any activities involved in training affect each of the systems to some extent. The interaction of systems should be kept in mind as a training program is planned. Each system must

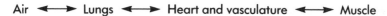

Air ⟷ Lungs ⟷ Heart and vasculature ⟷ Muscle

Fig. 5-1 The relationship between the lungs, the heart and circulation, and the metabolizing muscles.

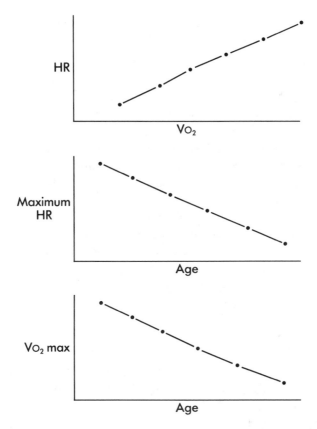

Fig. 5-2 A, The relationship between HR and V_{O_2}. **B,** The relationship between maximum HR and age. **C,** The relationship between V_{O_2}max and age.

be trained to function at its highest level possible while accommodating an individual's physical limitations.

An understanding of the normal response to exercise is a helpful foundation for training a disabled or deconditioned individual. Fig. 5-2 shows three graphs depicting the relationship among the heart, oxygen consumption, and age in normal persons. The three points brought out in these graphs will be even more important later in this chapter as we try to understand exercise prescription and responses to exercise testing.

Heart rate (HR) and oxygen consumption (V_{O_2}) in body tissue are linearly and directly related: HR increases proportionally to V_{O_2} (Fig. 5-2, *A*). This will be true throughout a progressively increasing work load until maximum exercise capacity is reached. At a maximum work load HR and V_{O_2} will plateau as cardiac output reaches its peak. HR and V_{O_2} will remain at this plateau even as work load increases, and the individual will soon stop exercising because of exhaustion.

Maximum HR and V_{O_2} are linearly and inversely related to age; that is, as age increases, the maximum HR and maximum V_{O_2} that can be achieved will decrease (Fig. 5-2, *B* and *C*). A 20-year-old individual may be able to achieve a maximum HR of approximately 200, but by the time this person is 60, his maximum HR will be approximately 160. Because of the relationship between HR and V_{O_2}, it is apparent that as age increases, the maximum ability to work decreases. The equation 220 − age is the most straightforward means of predicting maximum HR. Another formula, [210 − (age × 0.65) = maximum HR], allows for slightly greater accuracy. The value thus determined is not an absolute and should be considered only as a calculated prediction. An exercise stress test is the only means of confidently determining the maximum HR of an individual.

Many factors affect the actual limit of exercise tolerance, but the relationship between HR and age will always hold true. As a result an individual's functional capacity diminishes as he gets older. This decrease in maximum work capacity may be modified through training. Although they will not be able to work like they did when they were 25 years old, elderly people who are well conditioned will be able to perform at a higher level than their peers.

PREDICTING ABILITY AND DISABILITY

The term $V_{O_2}max$ is expressed in L/min or ml/kg/min and is the highest achievable extraction of oxygen by the body from the volumes of air breathed into the lungs. It is an indirect measure of total cellular metabolism in the body and is equated to the energy being expended or the work being done by the body. Two different terms can be used in reference to V_{O_2}. One is *predicted $V_{O_2}max$;* the other is *achieved $V_{O_2}max$.* Achieved $V_{O_2}max$ is an indication of functional capacity (ability) or the individual's level of fitness. Achieved $V_{O_2}max$, measured during a stress test, is the individual's ability to function in activities that require energy expenditure. V_{O_2} measurements that are less than maximum are called submax. V_{O_2} indicates the amount of energy required to perform the amount of work being done at that work load. Predicted $V_{O_2}max$ is based on studies conducted on individuals of the same gender and age. The more fit an individual is, the greater the likelihood she will achieve the maximum predicted V_{O_2}. A highly trained, world-class athlete may even exceed the maximum predicted V_{O_2}. But a sedentary or deconditioned patient will have an achieved $V_{O_2}max$ significantly less than the predicted maximum.

ARMSTRONG-WORKMAN NOMOGRAM

The Armstrong-Workman nomogram has been developed to aid in the determination of predicted Vo_2max in persons with normal lungs and in those with an obstructive pulmonary disorder (Fig. 5-3). The Vo_2max predicted from this nomogram for an individual with a pulmonary disorder is called the *adjusted Vo_2max*. This adjustment is necessary because a patient with a pulmonary disorder has a limit to his ventilatory abilities, as opposed to a cardiac limitation. Normally the limit to exertion exists in a component of the cardiovascular system, such as HR and stroke volume (SV).

No one is able to function at 100% of ability for any great length of time. The normal work capacity for an 8-hour occupational workday is between 25% and 40% of achieved Vo_2max. This information can be very useful when counseling individuals about occupations, leisure activities, and household chores (see Appendix D).

Percentages of achieved Vo_2max are also useful for exercise prescription in a training program. The prediction of Vo_2max is not intended to be a limit on ability but

For estimation of a predicted "normal" Vo_2 max and a predicted adjusted Vo_2 max.

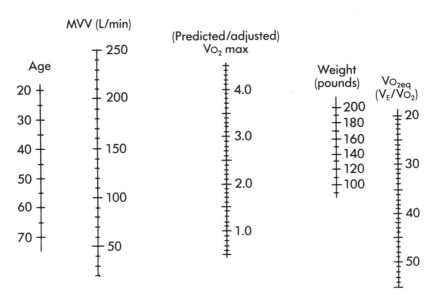

Fig. 5-3 The Armstrong-Workman nomogram, used for estimation of predicted "normal" Vo_2max and predicted "adjusted" Vo_2max. (Redrawn with permission. From Armstrong BW et al: Clinico-physiologic evaluation of physical working capacity in persons with pulmonary disease, Part I, Am Rev Respir Dis 93:97, 1966.)   *Continued.*

Example of an estimation of a predicted "normal" VO₂ max for a
60-year-old male weighing 170 pounds.

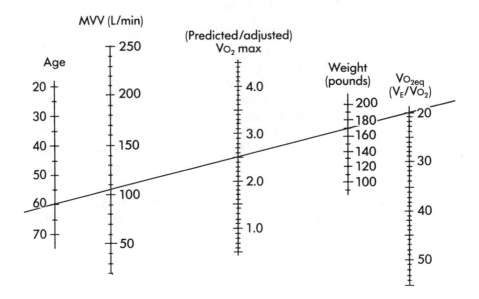

Example of an estimation of a predicted adjusted VO_2 max for
a 60-year-old male weighing 170 pounds suffering from COPD.
Measured MVV_{15} = 120 L/min, and a measured VO_{2eq} = 40 L/min.

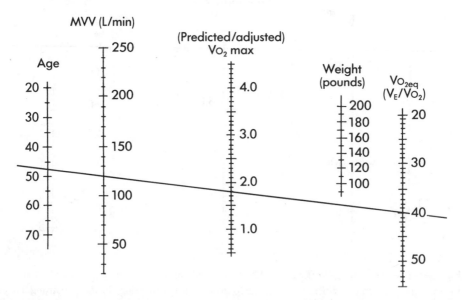

Fig. 5-3, cont'd. The Armstrong-Workman nomogram, used for estimation of predicted "normal" VO_2max and predicted "adjusted" VO_2max. (Redrawn with permission. From Armstrong BW et al: Clinico-physiologic evaluation of physical working capacity in persons with pulmonary disease, Part I, Am Rev Respir Dis 93:97, 1966.)

USE OF THE ARMSTRONG-WORKMAN
NOMOGRAM TO PREDICT NORMAL AND ADJUSTED Vo₂max

Normal Vo₂max

Identify the patient's age on the scale labeled *age* and the patient's weight on the scale labeled *weight*. Draw a line through these two points. The point at which this line intersects the scale labeled *Vo₂max* is the patient's predicted normal Vo₂max.

Adjusted Vo₂max

Identify the patient's measured MVV on the scale labeled *MVV* and the patient's measured ventilatory equivalent for O₂ at rest on the scale labeled $V_{eq}O_2$. Draw a line through these two points. The point at which this line intersects the scale labeled *Vo₂max* is the patient's predicted adjusted Vo₂max.*

*If the actual MVV has not been measured, an estimate can be made from the measured FEV₁ × 35. If the measured $V_{eq}O_2$ is not available, an approximate high normal value for $V_{eq}O_2$, 25-35, can be used. Use of either of these estimates will make the predicted adjusted value less accurate.

Table 5-1 Normal values for Vo₂max, resting Vo₂ and Vco₂, and RER

	Children (8 to 19 years old)		Adults (more than 20 years old)	
	Males	Females	Males	Females
Vo₂max	~50 ml O₂/min/kg	~45 ml O₂/min/kg	$[4.2 - (0.032 \times \text{age})]$ = Vo₂max expressed in L/min $[60 - (0.55 \times \text{age})]$ = Vo₂max expressed in ml/kg/min	$[2.6 - (0.014 \times \text{age})]$ = Vo₂max expressed in L/min $[48 - (0.37 \times \text{age})]$ = Vo₂max expressed in ml/kg/min
Vo₂	250 ml/min or ~3.5 ml/kg/min			
Vco₂	200 ml/min or ~2.8 ml/kg/min			
RER	200:250 (Vco₂:Vo₂) = 0.8			

a guideline for safety. Table 5-1 gives some normal values and equations for predicting Vo₂max, resting Vo₂, resting Vco₂, and respiratory exchange ratio (RER) Vco₂: Vo₂.

MET, Vco₂, AND RER

Frequently energy expenditure during various activities is expressed not in ml/min but as multiples of resting energy expenditure, called a metabolic equivalent (MET). MET is calculated by dividing Vo₂ during the activity by resting Vo₂. MET is a convenient measurement with many applications in exercise training and counseling (see Appendix D).

$$\mathrm{MET} = \frac{\text{Exercise } V_{O_2}}{\text{Resting } V_{O_2}}$$

V_{CO_2} is frequently measured along with V_{O_2} at rest or during exercise. V_{CO_2} is an indirect measure of cellular function because CO_2 is a primary by-product of metabolism. V_{CO_2} rises linearly and directly with an increasing work load. At maximum V_{O_2}, V_{CO_2} continues to rise as CO_2 diffuses into the bloodstream for removal by the lungs. In normal healthy individuals at sea level, hydrogen ions produced from various sources during metabolism, such as CO_2 and lactic acid in the blood, are the central stimulation for ventilation. The rate and volume of ventilation increases proportionally as the V_{CO_2} increases during exercise. The value V_{CO_2} is not useful by itself in exercise training but is used in other applications of indirect calorimetry.

RER is similar in concept to the respiratory quotient (RQ), and the two terms are often used interchangeably. RQ is the measured metabolism at the cellular level, whereas RER is determined by indirect measurement of V_{CO_2} and V_{O_2} in expired gas. Therefore RER is a reflection of cellular metabolism.

An indication of the efficiency of ventilation related to metabolism level is the ventilatory equivalent for O_2 and CO_2. The normal $V_{O_{2eq}}$ is 20 to 25 L of air per liter of O_2 consumed, that is, a resting ventilation of 5 L per resting V_{O_2} of 0.25 L. When a healthy person exercises, $V_{O_{2eq}}$ remains close to this value until the $V_{O_{2eq}}$ approaches maximum exercise capacity. As it approaches maximum effort, the ventilatory system is unable to increase output in response to the V_{CO_2} produced by the exercise. At this point the $V_{O_{2eq}}$ will increase as the respiratory system becomes less efficient. In a patient with a pulmonary disorder, $V_{O_{2eq}}$ can exceed 35 at rest and 50 or more at even submaximal work loads.

$V_{O_{2eq}}$ can help to identify the anaerobic threshold, the point during exercise at which the primary mechanism of metabolism changes from aerobic to anaerobic. It can be identified by graphing the values for V_{O_2}, V_{CO_2}, and minute ventilation (V_E), achieved during an exercise stress test, against time or work load. The point of departure from linearity for both VE and V_{O_2} marks the anaerobic threshold. This point can be useful when prescribing exercise, for instance, to limit stress during training sessions.

An important purpose of exercise testing is to determine functional capacity or to identify an objective work limit for an individual. Some individuals cannot perform a stress test, and often the facilities for testing are unavailable. A numeric value can be assigned to functional capacity from a description of the onset of symptoms during activity. Table 5-2 gives symptoms as they relate to observations and complaints from the patient and relates them to the probable achieved V_{O_2}max, for example, functional capacity. Table 5-2 can be valuable in treating extremely disabled individuals and

Table 5-2 Functional capacity

Subjective		Achieved V_{O_2}max
No limits, no symptoms	$\geqslant$7 METS	$\geqslant$21-24 ml/kg/min
Slight limitations, symptoms with heavy activity	5-6 METS	15-18 ml/kg/min
Marked limitations, symptoms with ordinary activity	3-4 METS	9-12 ml/kg/min
Discomfort at rest and during all activities	1-2 METS	3- 6 ml/kg/min

should be relied on only in situations in which stress testing is contraindicated or unavailable. Information such as functional capacity can be helpful during counseling (see Appendix D) and for pre-stress test determination of anticipated achieved V_{O_2}max. For example, a patient at level 4 in functional capacity (see Table 5-2) probably will have such a low maximal energy capacity that he will be unable to perform almost any activity without experiencing discomfort. This patient still can be educated and trained in self-care and perhaps can be strengthened. When motivated and placed on a well-designed program of ventilation retraining and strength training, the patient's ability may increase significantly.

DECONDITIONING IN DISABILITY

The patient with obstructive lung disease frequently falls into a downward spiral of diminishing activity. Because the patient is able to expend very little energy without experiencing symptoms, the effects of inactivity are progressively worsened. To minimize discomfort in breathing and to delay fatigue, many ADL are avoided. Activities that require the patient to exert physical effort may become sources of anxiety. Inactivity has a severe effect on the quality of life and the overall physical condition of the patient with COPD. Following are some of the nonspecific objectives that can be achieved through exercise training. They are reasonable objectives for the patient to try to achieve, but she should translate them into specific meaningful, and measurable objectives:
1. Increase functional capacity
2. Improve tolerance of ADL
3. Reduce sensitization to dyspnea
4. Improve ventilatory muscle strength
5. Improve arm and leg strength
6. Improve sense of well-being and self-esteem
7. Reduce somatic concern
8. Reduce fear of activities

Our bodies adapt physiologically to our lifestyle and the level of activity we maintain. These adaptations can be positive, for example, improvements in strength and endurance resulting from training, or negative, for example, the deconditioning

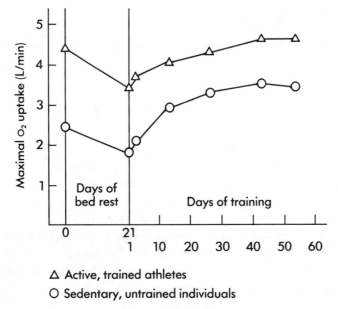

Fig. 5-4 Changes in Vo_2max in physically trained and sedentary individuals after bed rest and subsequent retraining. The top line illustrates Vo_2max in two trained individuals. The bottom line illustrates Vo_2max in three sedentary individuals. (Adapted from Saltin B et al: Response to exercise after bed rest and after training, Circulation 38, [suppl 7] Nov 1968.)

that results from prolonged bed rest and a sedentary lifestyle. This phenomenon is demonstrated graphically in Fig. 5-4. The study that produced this graph involved normal, healthy individuals, some of whom were physically trained (group A), some of whom were sedentary (group B). Each group's maximum Vo_2 was determined. Then each group was placed on strict bed rest for 2 weeks. Each individual was then retested to determine maximum Vo_2, and an 8-week training program designed to improve cardiopulmonary function was initiated.

The results showed marked deconditioning in both groups after the bed rest, as evidenced by a decrease in maximum Vo_2. Loss of muscle tone and general weakness were noted subjectively. Six weeks after the training program began, a significant improvement in maximum Vo_2 was evident. In group A, returning to the original baseline ability level required approximately 6 weeks, and little improvement over the baseline was noted. In group B, returning to this level also required approximately 6 weeks, but a significant improvement beyond it was noted as training continued.

EFFECTS OF INACTIVITY

Several points from this study can have important implications for the hospitalized patient. First, even short periods of strict inactivity can have a major effect on overall

---

EFFECTS OF INACTIVITY

Metabolism

Decreased metabolic rate, decreased protein catabolism, negative nitrogen balance, decubitus ulcers, imbalance of cellular electrolytes, and gastrointestinal hypomotility

Psychosocial

Decreased learning ability, decreased motivation to learn, decreased retention of new material, decreased problem-solving ability, exaggerated or inappropriate emotional reactions, perceptual and motor changes, and increased somatic concerns

Respiratory system

Decreased movement of secretions, decreased use of respiratory muscles, and development of microatelectasis and infection

Muscular system

Loss of normal muscle tone, decreased muscle efficiency, increased local muscle V_{O_2}, rapid onset of fatigue, and contracture

Cardiopulmonary system

Decreased cardiac output, venous stasis, thromboembolism, and pulmonary emboli

Skeletal system

Osteoporosis, reabsorption of calcium from the bone, and increased incidence of compression fractures

---

fitness and the ability to return to the level of work tolerated before inactivity. A 2-week hospitalization consisting of bed rest will result in a loss of functional capacity. Second, an individual's functional capacity is not static but is adaptive and is maintained at the level of activity or ability consistently demanded of the system. Third, the more sedentary or deconditioned an individual is initially, the greater the potential for improvement beyond a baseline ability level. In other words, an individual who begins a training program in relatively good condition will not experience as dramatic an improvement in ability and functional capacity as the individual who begins at a lower level of conditioning. Finally, the greatest improvement in functional capacity probably will be experienced in the first 6 weeks of the training period. After this time, effort will have to be increased steadily for improvement to continue.

The adaptation of the body to a lack of physical demands placed on it, as occurs during illness, is seen in almost every system of the body, particularly the muscular, cardiopulmonary, and skeletal systems. The general effects of inactivity are given in the box above.

Osteoporosis occurs in the skeletal system. This demineralization (loss of calcium, phosphorus, and nitrogen) contributes to malformation of the bone and increased incidence of compression fractures. Increased mineral intake is not the solution for the problem because the extra minerals will only be secreted in the urine. Weight-bearing mobility activities are the best method of preventing demineralization. The severely osteoporotic patient may experience a great deal of pain with weight-bearing activity; therefore a physical therapist skilled in rehabilitation techniques involving weight-bearing activities and familiar with pain management should be consulted.

Muscles experience atrophy and a loss of functional ability when subjected to long periods of disuse. The loss of strength in an immobilized muscle has been estimated to be approximately 10% to 15% per week. Muscle contracture results from loss of the muscular fibers' full range of shortening and lengthening abilities. The confinement of a muscle or joint in one position or within a limited range of motion is a chief cause of contracture of individual muscle groups. It is important that contracture be prevented in the intercostal muscles of the chest and other secondary muscles of ventilation. Physical therapy is vital to contracture prevention and should be initiated as early as possible.

Inactivity affects the cardiovascular system in three ways: orthostatic hypotension, increased work load for the heart, and formation of thrombi and emboli. Orthostatic hypotension is caused by a loss of muscle tone and subsequent pooling of blood in the peripheral venous system and a decrease in the efficiency of the neurovascular reflex. Changes in vascular resistance and hydrostatic pressure while lying supine cause the heart to work harder, resulting in increased HR and SV. Individuals subjected to prolonged bed rest have been known to have progressively increasing resting HR, approximately 0.5 beats per minute/day, and higher heart rates at low to moderate work loads than they did before they were confined to bed.

Thromboembolism formation is enhanced by venous stasis as a result of flaccid muscles and immobility. External pressure on the blood vessels may also contribute to thrombus formation. Prolonged or large amounts of pressure on a limb are always a concern in nursing care. The possible damage to the intima of the vessel may promote the laying down of plaque on the damaged site and may be a source of thrombus development. Frequent position changes are very important in preventing venous stasis. The routine changing of a patient's position every 2 hours may not be enough to promote comfort and ward off the effects of immobility because discomfort and local pressures can develop as often as every 2 minutes when the patient is in the recumbent position. Any exercise in bed should be of low intensity and progress slowly.

In general, muscle atrophy, loss of muscle function, and overall weakness lead to an increase in somatic concerns and poor motivation to pursue physical activities, which the patient perceives as strenuous. To prevent or interrupt the deconditioning effects of inactivity, a program of physical reconditioning and training should be implemented. Subjective and objective changes should be noted during training to provide a measure of improvement. These changes can also serve as a measure of patient compliance and a means of patient motivation.

PLANNING AN EXERCISE PROGRAM

Different aspects of training should be considered when planning an exercise program for the patient disabled by a pulmonary disorder. In general two aspects of training should be considered: strength training and endurance training.

"Specificity of training," the principle that training for one type of activity does not necessarily transfer to another type of activity, should be kept in mind when either strength training or endurance training is implemented. For example, in endurance training the only way to train to run faster or farther is to run. Training to swim farther or faster will not improve the runner's ability to achieve greater distances or speeds. This principle can also be applied to strength training. The muscles to be strengthened should be exercised according to the specific principles of training for those muscles. For example, general calisthenics will not increase leg strength as effectively as specific leg exercises will.

Strength-training activities are characterized as high in intensity but short in duration. Endurance-training activities are characterized as relatively low in intensity but high in duration. Generally an exercise with an intensity $\geq 90\%$ of the maximum ability of a specific muscle done in three sets of 10 to 15 repetitions each constitutes a strength-training exercise. When such training continues over a sufficient period of time, a specific muscle group is conditioned and strengthened. The more conditioned the individual is, the higher the intensity that will be required to achieve training of any muscle group.

Whenever possible, a specific muscle or group of muscles that require strengthening should be identified so that exercises designed for that muscle can be implemented. Some muscles to be considered are the hamstrings, quadriceps, deltoid, and abdominal muscles. From the physical assessment of the patient and the discussion of established goals, the specific muscles that require training can be identified and focused on during exercise. For example, to increase strength in his arms, the patient should be encouraged to lift a 1- or 2-pound weight 15 times or until his arm is fatigued, whichever comes first. He should rest and then repeat the exercise to complete three sets of 15 lifts. The type of lift to be performed will depend on the muscles that are the focus of the exercise. A curl strengthens the biceps. Lifting the arm from a resting position at the side to over the head strengthens the shoulder muscles, and curling from the wrist strengthens the forearm. The principle of using weights to strengthen muscles can also be applied during diaphragmatic/abdominal breathing retraining by placing a 2-pound weight on the abdomen during the breathing maneuver. Elaborate equipment is not necessary; a 1- or 2-pound can from the kitchen cupboard or an old plastic bottle filled with 1 or 2 pounds of sand can be used.

The patient should be encouraged to progress slowly through the training, especially through increasing intensities, to avoid undue stress on any particular muscle. There will probably be an accumulation of lactic acid in the muscle when training begins. The patient should be told that this accumulation will happen and that it may lead to soreness and some discomfort. Massaging the exercised area or moving the muscle group without resistance may improve circulation of blood through that area and enhance the buffering and removal of the lactic acid. As is necessary during all activities, proper breathing control must always be maintained. The strengthening aspect of an exercise, such as high intensity, may have to be sacrificed in favor of breathing control during the activity. The three key points in breathing control on p. 59 are always applicable for the patient with a pulmonary disorder.

TRAINING

Endurance-training activities focus on improving the function of the cardiopulmonary and cardiovascular systems. Improvements in these organ systems are not apparent in greater strength or muscle mass but in an increase in functional capacity, especially during ADL. Endurance training enables the heart and lungs to respond adequately to the demand for O_2 to be supplied to exercising muscles and for CO_2 to be removed from them.

Patients often require strength training before endurance training can begin. The little-used large-muscle groups, such as those in the legs, often are weak and must be strengthened before even a low-intensity endurance program is attempted. This may mean a 3- or 4-week period of intensive strength-training exercises. The patient should be able to demonstrate an improvement in the strength of muscle groups, as evidenced by increased ability and coordination, before progressing to endurance training.

Calisthenic and stretching exercises should be designed into a training program as a warm-up before the endurance activity. Some calisthenic exercises can also act as the endurance activity. (An example is given below.) Calisthenics also build coordination, which can benefit performance of other exercises and activities. Evidence of the endurance-building properties of calisthenics can be found in the use of calisthenics in the aerobic-exercise sessions many people participate in throughout the country. Table 5-3 gives two examples of how a series of calisthenic exercises can be planned, allowing for increasing intensity, as a training program for a patient. The exercises in a calisthenic-exercise program should be selected to allow the exercise session (exclusive of warm-up and cool-down) to take a total of 10 to 20 min. The patient may need to proceed very slowly at first. The emphasis in early exercise sessions should be on keeping the patient involved and moving while controlling her breathing for the entire exercise period. Later exercise sessions can focus on the quantity and quality of the calisthenics.

A number of exercises and the relative energy level into which each falls are given in Appendix G. These figures are broken into six levels of energy expenditure from the lowest to the highest. Those in levels I and II are appropriate for warm-up exercises but relatively inappropriate for endurance training (see Table 5-4). The

Table 5-3   Two sample exercise-session plans using calisthenic exercises*

Sample A		Sample B	
Intensity level	Exercise	Intensity level	Exercise
I	A	II	A
I	E	II	D
II	B	III	A
III	A	III	E
III	C	IV	B
IV	B	IV	D
V	B	V	A
V	E	V	C
VI	A	VI	C

*Illustrated in Appendix G.

intensity of the exercises in level VI can be appropriate for endurance training but may be too strenuous for some severely debilitated patients. The energy required to perform an exercise can be reduced by slowing the rate at which the exercise is done. Most patients can only tolerate an exercise program that can be completed in approximately 20 to 30 min, including time for warm-up and cool-down. The more disabled the patient, the slower her progress will be.

Although the intensity of endurance-training exercises is less than that of strength-training exercises, the time they require is significantly longer. Endurance activities require that the individual perform at ≥ 60% of maximum capacity for 20 to 30 min. Initially it may take several exercise sessions at the desired intensity level lasting less than 5 min each for some patients to accomplish a total of 20 minutes of endurance training. Although this is not "true" endurance training, it is a start, and the patient can eventually get to the point of sustained exercise (Fig. 5-5). Some patients will not be able to tolerate the intensity level of exercise for endurance training. In this case the emphasis should be on encouraging the patient to exercise at a level as high as possible while maintaining control and coordination of his breathing.

A primary characteristic of activities used for endurance training is that these activities can be sustained at a desired intensity for an extended period of time. Sports such as tennis, basketball, or volleyball are not true endurance activities. These activities do elicit high levels of energy expenditure. But the high-intensity exertion is quickly over, and a period of low intensity follows. Walking, swimming, bicycle riding, cross-country skiing, and jogging are examples of good activities for endurance training. These activities can be maintained at a desired intensity level under the control of the individual exercising for the amount of time necessary to benefit from the effects of training. It is unlikely that a patient with lung disease will jog or ski cross-country, but some individuals with early airway disease can try these activities.

The exercise method used for endurance training should be enjoyable. Enjoyment

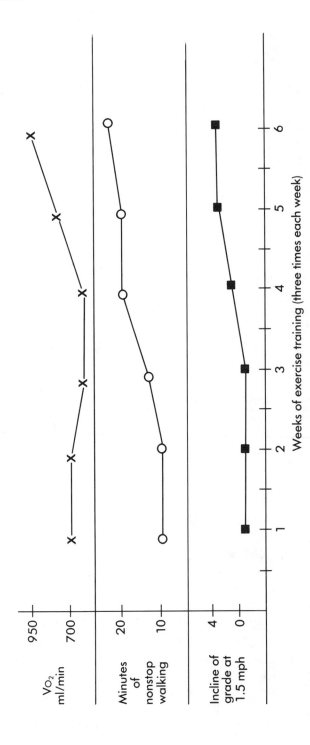

Fig. 5-5 Changes in a patient over 6 weeks of training.

and documented improvement will improve compliance with an endurance-training program. Slow progress is best to reduce injury and maximize benefits.

One training objective should be to improve coordination and mobility or ease of movement. Improved mobility of the extremities and the chest wall can improve their performance during activities such as walking. Stretching exercises for the chest and extremities should be included during warm-up and cool-down periods. Stretching can reduce strain during exercise and can improve the range of movement of the legs and arms. Patients with a restrictive lung disorder, such as a chest-wall deformity or splinting from pain or contractures, will find stretching and chest-mobility exercises helpful. A simple example of a chest-stretching exercise is the sigh. Slow, deep inhalation followed by slow, relaxed exhalation will move the ribs through the range of normal motion and keep the ligaments of the chest stretched out. Positive pressure, such as intermittent positive pressure breathing (IPPB) or manual ventilation, can be used for the paralyzed patient to stretch the thorax.

The technique used in walking can affect the energy required to carry out the activity. Often the patient who is weak from illness or injury will walk with a shuffle or in very short, "choppy" steps. This method of walking can double or triple the number of steps needed to cover a given distance, thus increasing the amount of energy needed. A patient who shuffles her feet while walking increases the resistance against which she must work to move her feet. Gait training teaches the patient to walk more efficiently. During gait training the patient learns to stretch out her stride, lift her feet while walking, and improve her balance.

VENTILATORY MUSCLE TRAINING

One aspect of training that has been of increasing interest recently is the training of inspiratory muscles. Several studies have shown improvement in patient performance of endurance activities simply by improving the function and strength of the patient's inspiratory muscles.

Two types of inspiratory training have been explored with patients: use of the inspiratory resistance devices (such as PFLEX™) and use of the maximum sustained ventilatory capacity (MSVC) breathing pattern. Both types of training emphasize improved strength of the ventilatory muscles.

With the inspiratory resistance device the patient begins training at a given level of resistance while inspiring. Resistance is controlled by the size of the opening through which the patient must inspire. The patient inspires through this device at the desired resistance for 10 minutes each day for 1 week. At the end of each week the resistance against which the patient must inspire is increased one level. As the patient progresses through the six levels of increasing resistance, the strength of his inspiratory muscles improves.

The MSVC maneuver is more complex, and the device is more technical and complicated. Essentially the patient performs an isocapnic hyperpnea (a rapid respiratory rate while maintaining a normal P_{CO_2}) for 15 min. The patient's respiratory rate is maintained at approximately 50% to 60% of MVV as determined in pulmonary-function testing. This maneuver is done under closely monitored conditions three times per week for 4 to 6 weeks. As the patient's work tolerance improves, the percentage of MVV at which he is ventilating can be increased to stimulate further training. This procedure requires monitoring of heart rate, blood pressure, and exhaled CO_2.

It is unclear whether exercising, such as walking, at an intensity that causes ventilation at greater than 50% of the resting MVV, like MSVC, results in the same ventilatory muscle training as the exercise performed at MSVC. Individuals using either method of ventilatory muscle training have shown improvement in the 12-minute-walk test as a measure of endurance. The 12-minute-walk test is the distance (for example, number of laps or feet) that the patient can walk in 12 minutes. If done before and after a training program, the test gives a fairly accurate indication of improvement in endurance. Patients using these training methods have also reported subjective improvements in physical ability and daily function.

THE EXERCISE PRESCRIPTION

The basic components of a program for reconditioning should be warm-up and cool-down routines lasting 10 min each, the exercise method to be performed, the specific level of exercise intensity, the duration of each exercise session, and the number of times each week the activity should be performed. This prescription format applies to both strength- and endurance-training programs. The box below shows the difference between endurance training and strength training. To ensure safety and proper training intensity, the patient must be trained to recognize signs of excessive exertion, such as a heart rate below or above the prescribed range or unusual muscle fatigue and soreness.

DIFFERENCES BETWEEN
ENDURANCE TRAINING AND STRENGTH TRAINING

Strength training involves a low number of repetitions of a high-intensity activity, such as lifting weights.

The patient performs three sets of 10 to 15 repetitions of an activity at 85% to 90% of the maximum capacity of the muscles being exercised.

Endurance training involves a high number of repetitions of a relatively low-intensity activity, such as walking.

The patient exercises nonstop for 20 to 30 min in a range of 60% to 80% of maximum HR.

In strength training the intensity of the exercise should be 85% to 90% of the patient's maximum achievable intensity. Although intensity can be tested using special isokinetic equipment, this is not usually done with patients; therefore, the patient's maximum ability is determined through trial and error. The duration of the high-intensity activity should be 10 to 15 repetitions of the specific motion or lift. In some instances this may be when fatigue is noticed. (If the patient is not able to perform the required 10 to 15 repetitions, the intensity is probably too high and should be reduced.) After a rest of 1 to 2 min the patient should repeat the 10 to 15 repetitions up to three times. The strength-training activity should imitate as much as possible the motion of normal daily activities, such as lifting, reaching, pulling, or pushing, and should take into account the patient's goals and the areas of weakness determined in the patient assessment.

During endurance activities, such as walking, the intensity must be greater than 60% but less than 80% of the patient's maximum HR. This intensity is required to achieve the classic training effect, a reduced HR at submaximal work loads. The heart rate is the best indicator of intensity and Vo_2 in endurance activities. Counting the pulse rate at the radial or brachial arteries for 15 seconds then multiplying this number by 4 will give a value for the HR in beats per minute.

The equations in the box below can be used to determine an intensity range for an endurance activity. It is difficult for anyone feeling his own pulse to obtain one precise number of beats per minute during exercise. By calculating a target range for his HR, stated as a number of beats every 15 or 30 seconds, the patient can monitor the intensity of exercise more easily.

The type of activity chosen for endurance training must be familiar to the patient. Compliance is increased by the enjoyment and convenience of the activity. Walking is perhaps the most widely used activity, but stair climbing and bicycle riding are also useful. A stationary bicycle may be best for patients who are unable to get outside to exercise and for those who require a controlled environment in which to exercise. It

---

TARGET HR AND INTENSITY FOR ENDURANCE TRAINING

Intensity for endurance training

60% to 80% of Vo_2max
  or
70% to 85% of maximum HR

Target HR for endurance training

Target HR = [% intensity(maximum HR − resting HR)] + resting HR
Examples: (.60[155 − 85]) + 85 = 127 BPM
           (.80[155 − 85]) + 85 = 141 BPM
           Target HR = 127-141 BPM or 32-35 BP15 seconds

LAP-TIME EQUATION

Distance (in feet) to be walked $\times$ 0.6818 = number of seconds per lap at 1 mph

Divide the number of seconds per lap at 1 mph by the speed (in mph) needed to achieve the target HR. (This speed is determined most easily by walking on a treadmill while monitoring HR.) This calculation will yield the number of seconds in which the distance must be walked to achieve the desired target HR.

Example: (220 ft.) $\times$ 0.6818 = 150 seconds per lap at 1 mph
(150 seconds per lap at 1 mph) divided by 2 mph = 75 seconds per lap to achieve the desired intensity of HR

---

may also be the best exercise method for all patients during inclement weather. The patient must be trained to monitor heart rate during any type of activity to ensure that it is within the target training range. Control and coordination of breathing must be maintained at all times during the endurance activity. Considerable practice may be necessary before actual endurance training can begin. Several activities are strenuous enough to be effective for endurance training: walking, jogging, swimming, bicycling, and doing aerobic calisthenics. Whatever the activity selected, the patient must be able to maintain it at a designated intensity for the required duration. Activities such as tennis, golf, or bowling, although enjoyable, do not meet these requirements and should not be substituted as a training activity.

Walking is the most practical, safest, and widely used endurance-training activity. The lap-time equation in the box above is an alternative method for determining and monitoring the intensity of a walking session and for monitoring progress over time. The patient can use it to calculate the number of seconds required to walk a known distance at 1 mph. This information can be very useful during early exercise sessions, especially if the patient is not being monitored closely by trained personnel. If the patient is walking a known distance, such as the length of a hallway, the time required to complete the activity can serve as a measure of achievement of a sufficient level of exertion.

The patient should perform strength and endurance activities every other day. The day between the exercise days allows the body to recover from the exertion, for example, by allowing built-up lactic acid to dissipate. This recovery period is a necessary part of training. Exercising more frequently than every other day, especially early in the training program, does not allow the body to recover and can demotivate the patient. The schedule described in the box on p. 91 allows the patient to recover adequately and prevents undue stress while the patient is achieving training goals. Following this schedule will result in improved endurance over a period of 4 to 8 weeks.

———— **FREQUENCY AND DURATION OF ENDURANCE TRAINING** ————

Frequency—Minimum of three times per week, with a day of rest between exercise days
(Monday, Wednesday, Friday, Sunday, Tuesday, Thursday, Saturday, Monday, etc.)
Duration*—Minimum of 20 to 30 min of exercise at the proper intensity

*To achieve the necessary duration of activity early in the training program, exercise sessions may be divided into three 10-min sessions or four 5-min sessions in the target HR range.

MEASURING IMPROVEMENT

The patient needs to be made aware that there will be soreness and perhaps a temporary increase in pulmonary symptoms, such as fatigue, SOB, and sputum production, at the beginning of the exercise program. As the exercise program progresses, some medications may need to be adjusted because of the change in the patient's metabolism. Although the classic training effect is not frequently seen in COPD patients, an improvement in their functional ability, especially their ability to perform ADL, has been noted. It is imperative that the plan of exercise reconditioning be individualized to accommodate each patient's needs, goals, and interests. These plans should be designed with the input of a physician knowledgeable in pulmonary disease and in the principles of exercise training.

Studies conducted to determine the improvement of the patient with COPD after exercise training have generally shown no measurable changes in pulmonary or cardiovascular function. Pulmonary function results, Vo_2max, and other parameters do not improve significantly from pre-training values after an exercise program. But the patient can do more, feels better, and can function at a higher level than before exercise training. Following are some of the suggested mechanisms of improvement for the COPD patient participating in an exercise-training program:

Increased motivation

Desensitization to dyspnea

Improved mechanical efficiency

Improved endurance of limb muscles

Improved endurance of ventilatory muscles

Motivation is certainly a key element. As the patient attempts activities and finds that he is able to do them, he wants to try to do more. The patient gains confidence as he learns to control his breathing instead of letting it control him. The desensitization to dyspnea that results from increased endurance is vital to breathing control during activities and difficult situations. Every person experiences dyspnea at some point during strenuous exertion, but the patient with a pulmonary disorder is frequently oversensitized to it and may take it as a sign of the limit to his ability. If an individual undergoing training were to stop at the first sign of dyspnea, the benefits of training would never be achieved.

Improved neuromuscular coordination, mechanical efficiency, and limb strength all contribute to the overall improvement in the ability to tolerate work. As arms and legs get stronger, fatigue is less likely to occur with minor exertion, and the patient is able to lift, reach, pull, or push with greater ease. The strength and efficiency of the ventilatory muscles increases. As a result less energy is expended in breathing, allowing the individual to expend the energy in other activities.

Routine follow-up allows for timely modification of a training program and an improvement in patient compliance. At some follow-up sessions the patient's strength and/or endurance can be assessed to verify any improvement. Also, follow-up visits allow the program to be tailored to meet individual needs even better and prevent overtraining or training at inappropriate times, such as while the patient is fighting a chest cold.

USE OF METS TABLES

Knowledge of tables of metabolic energy expenditures or METS for various activities is useful in counseling patients and planning a training program. This counseling may be in an occupation, in exercise training or leisure activities, or in performance of ADL. MET tables are helpful in identifying activities that will probably prove too strenuous for a patient and, therefore, should be avoided. The three tables listed in Appendix D give a sample of metabolic expenditure for occupational activities, leisure activities, and ADL.

Generally an occupational activity that requires greater than 40% of an individual's Vo_2max (functional capacity in METS) will prove too strenuous to be sustained for an 8-hour workday. Leisure activities and ADL will usually be performed at between 20% and 40% of the patient's functional capacity. Activities requiring energy expenditure above this point will probably prove too strenuous. To judge the maximum level at which an individual can function comfortably, it is best to have functional capacity measured through indirect calorimetry during an exercise stress test. However, if this

Table 5-4 The relationship between MET levels of an activity and the activity's value in endurance training*

MET level	Value in endurance training
1-2	Not strenuous enough for endurance training but useful for general conditioning if person is very deconditioned
3-4	Dynamic exercise, possibly useful in endurance training for very deconditioned person
5-6	Effective in endurance training for most normal persons
>7	Excellent endurance training. Caution should be used not to exceed target HR for training

*The MET tables in Appendix D suggest specific activities.

test is not available, a predicted maximum or an adjusted predicted maximum can be determined by using the Armstrong-Workman nomogram. The energy-expenditure levels predicted for each activity should be used as a guide for suggesting activity limits. The "true" ability of the COPD patient must be determined subjectively by the patient and measured objectively through testing. Table 5-4 gives a relationship between the MET level for an activity and the value of the activity as a method of endurance training.

BIBLIOGRAPHY
Physiology

Alpert JS et al: Effects of physical training on hemodynamics and pulmonary function at rest and during exercise in patients with chronic obstructive pulmonary disease, Chest 66(6):647-651, 1974.

Astrand P and Rodahl K: Textbook of work physiology, ed 2, New York, 1977, McGraw-Hill, Inc.

Belman MJ and Kendregan BA: Physical training fails to improve ventilatory muscle endurance in patients with chronic obstructive pulmonary disease, Chest 81(4):440-443, 1982.

Belman MJ and Sieck GC: The ventilatory muscles: fatigue, endurance and training, Chest 82(6):761-766, 1982.

Braun SR, Fregosi R, and Reddan WG: Exercise training in patients with COPD, Postgrad Med 71(4): 163-173, 1982.

Ingjer F and Stromme SB: Effects of active, passive or no warm-up on the physiological response to heavy exercise, Eur J Appl Physiol 40:273-282, 1979.

Jones NL, Jones G, and Edwards RHT: Exercise tolerance in chronic airway obstruction, Am Rev Respir Dis 103:477-491, 1971.

Jones NL: Pulmonary gas exchange during exercise in patients with chronic airway obstruction, Clin Sci 31:39-50, 1966.

Karvonen MJ, Kentala E, and Mustala O: The effects of training on heart rate: a longitudinal study, The Institute of Occupational Health, Helsinki, pp 307-315, 1957.

Knowlton RG, Miles DS, and Sawka MN: Metabolic responses of untrained individuals to warm-up, Eur J Appl Physiol 40:1-5, 1978.

Medical Center, University of Nebraska: Pulmonary rehabilitation medical manual, Omaha, 1976.

Olson EV, editor: The hazards of immobility, Am J Nurs 67(4):R-02, 1967.

Pardy RL et al: Inspiratory muscle training compared with physiotherapy in patients with chronic airflow limitation, Am Rev Respir Dis 123:421-425, 1981.

Schaanning J: Ventilatory and heart rate adjustments during submaximal and maximal exercise in patients with chronic obstructive lung disease, Scand J Respir Dis 57:63-72, 1976.

Smith EL and Serfass RC, editors: Exercise and aging: the scientific basis, pp 11-17 and 89-120, Hillside, NJ, 1980, Enslow Publishers.

Sonne LJ and Davis JA: Increased exercise performance in patients with severe COPD following inspiratory resistive training, Chest 81(4):436-439, 1982.

Spiro SG et al: An analysis of the physiological strain of submaximal exercise in patients with chronic obstructive bronchitis, Thorax 30:415-425, 1975.

Wasserman K and Whipp BJ: Exercise physiology in health and disease, Am Rev Respir Dis 112:321-351, 1975.

Testing

Armstrong BW et al: Clinico-physiologic evaluation of physical working capacity in persons with pulmonary disease, Part I, Am Rev Respir Dis 93:90-99, 1966.

Armstrong BW et al: Clinico-physiologic evaluation of physical working capacity in persons with pulmonary disease, Part II, Am Rev Respir Dis 93:223-233, 1966.

Brown HV, Wasserman K, and Whipp BJ: Strategies of exercise testing in chronic lung disease, Bull Eur Physiopathol Resp 13:409-423, 1977.

Jones NL: Exercise testing in pulmonary evaluation: rationale, methods and the normal respiratory response to exercise, N Engl J Med 293(11):541-544, 1975.

Jones NL: Exercise testing in pulmonary evaluation: clinical applications, N Engl J Med 293(13):647-650, 1975.

Wasserman K, editor: Supplement: exercise testing in the dyspneic patient, Am Rev Respir Dis 129(2), 1984.

Training

Belman MJ: Exercise physiology and its application in the training of patients with chronic obstructive pulmonary disease, City of Hope Q 8(3):3-5, 1979.

Belman MJ and Mittman C: Ventilatory muscle training improves exercise capacity in chronic obstructive pulmonary disease patients, Am Rev Respir Dis 121:273-280, 1980.

Belman MJ and Wasserman K: Exercise training and testing in patients with chronic obstructive pulmonary disease, Basics of RD 10(2):1-6, 1981.

Chester E et al: Multi-disciplinary treatment of chronic pulmonary insufficiency, Chest 72(6):695-702, 1977.

Degre S, Sobolski J, and Degre-Coustry C: Controversial aspects of physical training in patients with COPD, Practical Cardiology 37-45, Jan 1979.

Leith DE and Bradley M: Ventilatory muscle strength and endurance training, J Appl Physiol 41(4): 508-516, 1976.

May DF, Pilbeam SP, and Kenny WR: A modified exercise prescription for a patient with severe COPD, J Med Assoc Ga 71:703-706, Oct 1982.

Mertens DJ, Shephard RJ, and Kavanagh T: Long-term exercise therapy for chronic obstructive lung disease, Respiration 35:96-107, 1978.

Pierce AK et al: Response to exercise training in patients with emphysema, Arch Intern Med 113:78-86, Jan 1964.

Sobush D, Dunning M, and McDonald K: Exercise prescription components for respiratory muscle training: past, present and future, Respir Care 30(1):34-42, 1985.

Unger KM, Moser KM, and Hansen P: Selection of an exercise program for patients with chronic obstructive pulmonary disease, Heart Lung 9(1):68-76, 1980.

Weiss RA and Karpovich PV: Energy cost of exercises for convalescents, Arch Phys Med 28:447-454, 1947.

CHAPTER **6**

Medication and diet in treatment of pulmonary disorders

IMPORTANCE OF MEDICATION

Few areas of the health care plan for a patient can have a more dramatic effect on treatment than the medications prescribed by the physician. The physiologic effect of medication is not the only important factor in treatment; the method of administration and patient compliance with the prescribed schedule also play important parts in treatment. When medications are taken as prescribed, the level at which the patient performs ADL can be improved. The physician is concerned with the use of appropriate medication and dosages for the disease. As decisions are made about medications, it is important that the physician be made aware of any variation in dosage. Missing a day of taking the medication, forgetting to take a dose, or using a generic medication instead of the name brand can affect the monitoring of prescribed medications, drug interactions, and therapeutic effectiveness.

A written schedule for taking medications can be very helpful for the patient and her family. To minimize difficulty in following a medication schedule, the patient's lifestyle must be considered when the schedule is created. The schedule can help the physician and the patient communicate about the prescribed medications. Unfortunately many patients talk about being discharged from an acute-care facility with a long list of pills or treatments and an inadequate explanation of them and their effects. This lack of information is a chief cause of poor compliance with medication schedules and programs of self-care.

The patient and her family need to understand *why* a medication or treatment is prescribed. They should also understand *how* and *when* to administer medications and treatments. The discussion should include any precautions to be aware of and the actions and potential side effects of each medication. The need to discuss these three aspects of medications and therapy is greater if equipment or unique conditions are involved in administration of the medication, but they should still be discussed for "routine" medication administration. If the patient and family can repeat all instructions, follow the written schedule, and demonstrate techniques involved in the prescribed therapy, the likelihood of a successful program is improved.

Because cost is a major consideration in health care, the physician and the patient should discuss the issue of using generic vs. brand-name medications. Generic drugs carry the chemical (pharmacopoeia) name of the medication, and the companies that produce them are not identified. Essentially, generic and brand-name medications are identical, but a physician may have a reason for preferring that the patient use the brand name. This preference should be discussed with the patient. The physician may have had a favorable experience treating other patients with a certain brand of medication, and the prescribed medication may not have a generic equivalent. Generic drugs are usually less expensive than brand-name drugs. The high cost of medications and treatments can contribute to a lack of willingness to comply with the care program. By using generic and other lower-cost medications, the economic factors contributing to poor compliance can be minimized.

COMPLIANCE WITH PRESCRIBED MEDICATIONS AND THERAPY

A patient who is complying with her prescribed therapeutic regimen is willing to adhere to all aspects of the health care plan. The care plan for the patient will be made up of various treatments, exercises, medications, and scheduled activities, such as visits to the physician. It cannot be a foregone conclusion that a patient will comply with all aspects of self-care without guidance and follow-up from the health-care team. Compliance can be improved by creating a health care plan that is easy to adhere to, fits the patient's lifestyle, and provides for accountability.

Many factors can contribute to poor compliance. The health-care team should watch for them and deal with them as soon as they are recognized. The severity of the disorder, previous hospital experiences, and the age or gender of the patient do not seem to affect the patient's willingness to comply, but they may affect the patient's ability to comply. A common influence on compliance is an adverse or unpleasant reaction to a medication, such as Cushing syndrome, which results from the prolonged use of steroids. Nausea, tremors, headaches, and listlessness are frequent complaints from patients taking the routine medication given for a pulmonary disorder. It may take a period of weeks or months for a patient to adjust to a medication. It is important that the patient communicate with the physician during this early part of his care plan. Adverse reactions to medication may be caused by a single medication, its dosage, or the interaction of one medication with another. The physician must be aware of the patient's level of compliance, such as whether he takes his medication in the prescribed dose and at the right time, to make appropriate adjustments to the prescribed therapy.

Self-administration of over-the-counter medications can be a major contributing factor to adverse reactions to medication and may complicate the identification of a source for these reactions. The physician should be notified that the patient is taking over-the-counter medications.

A major factor in poor compliance is confusion about the prescribed regimen for taking medications. It is not unusual for a patient to be taking six or more medications for pulmonary or other medical problems. The addition of respiratory treatments, exercises, and other aspects of a respiratory care plan can contribute to a very complicated schedule of self-care. Each medication or treatment has unique traits that add to a complicated body of information for the patient. Incomplete or unclear instructions, such as conflicting information about medications and jargon used to explain the material, contribute to confusion and poor compliance. Well-written instructions and a written medication or therapy schedule can be important in preventing or correcting confusion and poor compliance.

Some patients have a personality that makes them more compliant with a planned therapy program than others. A patient who is asymptomatic or who has an independent type of personality tends to be less compliant than patients who are symptomatic or who have a dependent type of personality. An independent patient who is experiencing severe symptoms has a tendency to comply with the prescribed care at least until the symptoms are relieved. At this point unless further follow-up and reinforcement are provided, the patient may not continue the care plan until further exacerbation is experienced. The dependent patient who is asymptomatic may also have trouble complying with a care program. The health-care team should watch that some patients do not overcomply with the plan of care and therapy.

Several methods have been found to be helpful in increasing patient compliance with a program of care. Foremost among them is the development of a strong relationship between the patient and the members of the health-care team. The physician is the key figure in this relationship; however, therapists, nurses, and other health-care professionals involved with the patient on a regular basis also have important roles to play. A structured educational program can also improve compliance. Such a program should include all members of the health-care team, and instructions should be given to the patient in writing that is simple and clear. Ambivalence or disagreements among team members must be avoided. Schedules, charts, and check-off sheets are helpful reminders for proper administration of medications and treatments.

Self-diagnosis and self-treatment of symptoms, which can lead to complications, can be reduced if health-care practitioners are accessible to the patient. It is important that the patient know whom to contact when symptoms arise, as well as when and how to contact this person. Decreasing the waiting time to speak with or see a physician or to receive therapy as an outpatient can improve a patient's willingness to comply with and participate in his own health care.

BASIC INFORMATION ABOUT COMMON PULMONARY MEDICATIONS
Bronchodilators

The primary action of a bronchodilator is to relax contracted smooth muscle in the airway. This relaxation can lead to relief of bronchospasm and SOB and reduction of wheezing. Some bronchodilators also contain anti-inflammatory agents, which contribute to an increase in the lumen of the airway by reducing the edema in inflammation.

Bronchodilators are most effective when taken according to a regular schedule that maintains a specific amount of the medication in the blood. Bronchodilators may be taken as a suppository, as an inhalant, by injection, and orally as a pill or elixir. Many different bronchodilators are available. Some have a longer duration of action and fewer side effects throughout the body than others. Inhaled bronchodilators have a topical effect, acting directly on the airways. A common method of medication administration in pulmonary disorders, inhaled bronchodilators act quickly and have fewer systemic side effects but may not last as long as bronchodilators administered orally.

Upset stomach and loss of appetite are common side effects of bronchodilators, especially when administered orally. Other common side effects are an increase in heart rate, a "jittery" or nervous feeling, tremors in the extremities, and headache. If the patient experiences any of these side effects, she should mention them to her physician.

Steroids

Steroids are given for their anti-inflammatory actions and for maintaining tone in the muscles of the airway. Increased healing, improved response to other therapy, reduced number and severity of symptoms, elevated mood, and a general feeling of well-being are also attributed to these medications. The action of steroids is not well understood.

Management of steroids can be a difficult task. A delicate balance between their positive and negative effects is required. The normal production of corticosteroids by the adrenal glands can be suppressed through the administration of steroids. Most physicians prefer to use steroids only for a limited time, but this is not possible for some patients. The patient must be removed from oral steroids slowly and gradually, and the removal should be monitored closely. The gradual nature of the removal can make the medication schedule during steroid removal very complicated, for example, five pills each day for 1 week, then four pills each day for 1 week, etc. Whenever oral steroids are taken, all dosages should be administered in the morning with food. Steroids can also be inhaled to act topically in the lungs. When taken with an inhaled bronchodilator, the steroid should be taken after waiting 10 minutes from the inhalation of a bronchodilator. The patient should be urged to rinse her mouth well after inhaling the steroid to prevent buildup of *Candida* in the mouth.

Because a patient taking steroids may feel that she has more energy than before, she may overextend herself. This overextension of abilities should be avoided. Another effect of steroids can be a weight gain, primarily from fluid retention. The patient is easily bruised, and with extended use the redistribution of fat deposits in the body may give the patient a "moon face" appearance. It is also possible for steroids to mask symptoms of pulmonary disease. For example, infections may not be noticed as quickly as they would if steroids were not being used, and SOB from an exacerbation of the disease takes longer to manifest itself. The normal production of corticosteroids by the adrenal glands can be suppressed when taking steroids. Stomach ulcers, fluid retention, fungal infections (especially oral infections with the use of inhaled steroids), and reduced function of the immunologic system are all side effects of steroid use. Use of inhaled steroids can reduce the incidence of many of the systemic side effects mentioned above. Inhaled steroids are also useful for weaning a patient from oral steroids.

Cromolyn sodium

Cromolyn sodium prevents the degranulation of the mast cell and the release of histamine, slow-reacting substance of anaphylaxis (SRSA), and other mediators and is useful only as a prophylactic. These mediators can induce bronchospasm, edema, and inflammation of the airways, especially in allergic asthma. Once the symptoms of an allergic attack of asthma, such as wheezing and SOB, has begun, cromolyn sodium is not beneficial but instead can complicate the problem.

When administered regularly, cromolyn sodium maintains the integrity of the mast cell, and the mediators are not released. It is administered through inhalation, usually four times each day. Like a steroid, cromolyn sodium is most effective when inhaled after the bronchodilator has been administered. This order of administration aids in the deposition of cromolyn sodium in the airways. Cromolyn sodium is a topically acting medication. Some of its side effects are coughing, wheezing, rash, itching, and nausea.

Expectorants

The benefit of an expectorant in treating a pulmonary disorder is unclear. There may be an increase in the mucociliary escalator as a mechanism for moving secretions in the airway toward the mouth. Some studies have reported stimulation of mucus production, an increase in the liquidity of mucus, and decreased viscosity. The purpose of an expectorant is to facilitate removal of secretions from the airways.

The best expectorant is water, which has almost no side effects and is rapidly absorbed into the pulmonary system. A regular regimen of water consumption at 1.5 quarts per day should be instituted and must continue before it can have a beneficial effect. Fluid intake, especially water, should be scheduled between meals to prevent abdominal distension and breathing difficulty while eating. Other expectorants can be found in pill form, in elixirs, or in drops that can be placed in drinks. Some of the most commonly used expectorants other than water are super-saturated potassium iodide (SSKI) and glyceryl guaiacolate (guaifenesin).

Reported reactions to the iodide in SSKI include allergic reactions, swelling of salivary glands, rhinitis, skin rash, and nausea. The side effects of these medications and the lack of evidence of their effectiveness may outweigh their usefulness.

Antibiotics

It is difficult to imagine health care today without antibiotics. The action of antibiotics is to destroy a disease-causing organism or suppress its growth. Antibiotics affect bacteria, not viruses, so, for example, they are not useful in treating the common cold and flu. Numerous antibiotics are available. They are usually prescribed according to the organism causing the disease. A broad-spectrum antibiotic, effective against a wide number of common bacteria, may be prescribed as a prophylaxis, for example, when respiratory infections occur frequently.

Antibiotics should be used carefully, and use should be monitored by a physician. Some bacteria have developed resistance to certain antibiotics, which had initially been effective against them. Whenever antibiotics are prescribed, the full dosage, for example, 30 pills, should be taken as directed. Adhering to the duration of the prescription, such as 7 to 10 days, helps prevent development of bacteria that are resistant to the antibiotic. Each antibiotic has unique precautions. Some must be taken with food. Others should not be taken with dairy products. In general it is best to administer the medication about 30 minutes before meals to improve its absorption into the body. To maximize the effectiveness of the medication, explicit information about its effects and precautions must be provided to the patient.

The side effects of antibiotics are different for each medication and each patient. Patients taking antibiotics often complain of nausea and diarrhea, and some patients become sensitive to sunlight.

Diuretics

Some patients, usually those who have heart disease along with the pulmonary disorder, need a diuretic. The primary action of the diuretic is to help the kidneys excrete fluids from the body, which reduces the work of the heart, blood pressure, and ankle and leg edema. The loss of fluid also lowers the patient's body weight and allows for improved mobility and lower work of breathing.

In general, diuretics are taken during the day—never in the evening or before retiring for the night. The patient's fluid intake may need to be restricted while he is taking these medications, and a physician will need to monitor the patient carefully. If the patient produces excessive pulmonary secretions, a careful balance must be achieved between fluid intake (to prevent thickened mucus) and dosage of the diuretic (to reduce ankle swelling).

A frequent problem associated with the use of diuretics is loss of potassium, which can lead to weakness, leg cramps, and occasional dizziness. Potassium supplements can be taken, but they are usually poorly tolerated because of the upset stomach and "iron" taste of the medication. A diet that includes some of the many foods high in potassium, such as bananas and oranges, is usually sufficient to prevent a potassium deficiency. The patient should have his serum potassium level determined occasionally to ensure that a low potassium level does not become a problem.

VACCINATIONS FOR FLU AND PNEUMONIA

Vaccinations should be administered routinely to any patient with a pulmonary disorder. Immunization is available for pneumococcal pneumonia and viral infections such as influenza, both of which have serious consequences for pulmonary patients. Although inoculation does not prevent the patient from getting the infection, it reduces the incidence and severity of infection. The flu vaccine is usually administered in the fall of each year, but the pneumonia vaccination is usually administered only once in a lifetime. Common side effects of vaccination are soreness at the sight of the injection and flu-like symptoms (occasional fever and general weakness).

OXYGEN

Oxygen is a drug that, like other medications, can be administered to a patient only by prescription from a physician. Oxygen is administered at a specific flow rate, such as a number of L/min. The required amount can be determined by testing ABG. The greatest benefit of oxygen therapy is seen when the gas is administered 24 hours a day. The use of oxygen intermittently, such as for a few hours a day or only during periods of SOB, is inappropriate. Some patients require that the number of L/min administered during activities such as exercise sessions be changed from the number given at rest. Changes in the prescribed number of liters should never be made without the physician's knowledge. The type of equipment used in oxygen therapy, the characteristics of the gas, and its application are covered in Chapter 7.

SCHEDULES FOR TAKING MEDICATIONS AT HOME

It is important to establish rapport with the patient before writing a medication schedule for her. The patient contributes to the schedule by making it practical. This participation can enhance the patient's confidence in her ability to adhere to the schedule. The health-care practitioner making the schedule should inquire about the patient's past compliance with prescribed medications and treatments, paying particular attention to any problems that may have contributed to a lack of compliance.

The patient can acquire knowledge of her medication through a question-and-answer session on specific medication. If any misinformation or lack of knowledge has been noted, it can be corrected at this time. During this session the patient's lifestyle and ADL, such as work schedule, hobbies, and eating and sleeping habits, should be considered.

Bronchodilators should be administered before the most active periods of each day. The purpose of such a schedule is to allow for maximum benefit from the bronchodilator during those times when it is probably needed most. To produce the maximum effect with minimum side effects, oral and aerosolized bronchodilators should be scheduled so that the onset and duration of each is complementary to the other. The patient should be informed of the amount of time normally required for bronchodilators to act, such as peak blood levels. If nausea, lack of appetite, or other symptoms are noted, the probable source of the problem may then be easier to identify. It may help to schedule the bronchodilators at mealtime if these problems persist. Adequate fluid intake (eight to ten glasses per day) should be included in the schedule. Diuretics should be taken only in the morning or early afternoon to prevent disruptions of sleep to urinate.

Generally antibiotics should be administered approximately 30 min before meals to promote better absorption. Some antibiotics must be taken with food. Others require that certain types of food be avoided. For example, tetracycline should not be taken with dairy products. The package insert with the medication provides this information. It is usually convenient to schedule administration of antibiotics at the time of fluid intake.

When a patient is receiving inhaled steroids and an aerosolized bronchodilator, administration of the inhaled steroid should follow administration of bronchodilator by at least 10 min. Administration of cromolyn sodium should also follow administration of an aerosolized bronchodilator by 10 min. The total dose of oral steroids should be administered at one time, usually in the morning.

A patient's medication schedule should not require that the patient take a medication or administer a treatment at every waking hour of the day. Such a schedule would not promote compliance or allow the patient to lead a normal life. The health-care practitioner making the schedule should be sensitive to the patient's needs to ensure that the schedule is not burdensome. Input from the patient when the schedule is made enhances patient compliance with the program when she is away from the staff's direct supervision.

A medication schedule like the sample in Fig. 6-1 is patient-oriented and would be easy to follow. Note the lack of jargon. The patient's usual time of rising and going to bed, eating meals, and performing other ADL should be determined. The schedule should be integrated as much as possible into the patient's present lifestyle. Finally the person making the schedule should ask himself: "Would I follow this schedule if it were mine?" If not, it should be redone with input from a physician. Ways to improve organization and perhaps eliminate some of the treatments, exercises, or medications should be sought.

Following are the prescribed medications and dosages for a hypothetical patient.

Anhydrous theophylline (Theo Dur): 300 mg bid

Metaproterenol sulfate (Alupent): 2 puffs qid

Furosemide (Lasix): 5 mg bid

Beclomethasone dipropionate (Vanceril): 2 puffs qid

Digoxin: 0.25 mg qid

Tetracycline: †

The patient should drink one full glass of water at each scheduled medication time. While avoiding caffeine and alcohol, the patient should drink approximately 10 glasses of liquid per day.

The following chart is for a hypothetical patient who reports rising at 7 AM and retiring at 10 PM. The patient would record the date and place a check mark in the box beside each dose after it has been administered.

Time	Medication	Date:							
7 AM	Anhydrous theophylline (1 tablet)								
	Metaproterenol sulfate (2 puffs)								
	Beclomethasone dipropionate (2 puffs)*								
	Furosemide (1 tablet)								
	Digoxin (1 tablet)								
11 AM	Metaproterenol sulfate (2 puffs)								
	Beclomethasone dipropionate (2 puffs)*								
3 PM	Metaproterenol sulfate (2 puffs)								
	Beclomethasone dipropionate (2 puffs)*								
7 PM	Anhydrous theophylline (1 tablet)								
	Metaproterenol sulfate (2 puffs)								
	Beclomethasone dipropionate (2 puffs)*								
	Furosemide (1 tablet)								
10 PM	Metaproterenol sulfate (2 puffs)‡								

Comments and reminders:

*Drug should be administered 10 minutes after metaproterenol sulfate with 1 minute between puffs.

†One pill should be administered four times each day only when sputum turns green. Drug should not be taken with dairy products, and the patient's physician should also be called.

‡Drug should be administered only if needed during the night.

Fig. 6-1 Sample medication table for hypothetical patient.

OVER-THE-COUNTER MEDICATIONS

Self-medication with products that can be purchased from any pharmacy is a common practice for patients suffering from symptoms of a pulmonary disorder. Television advertisements promise a restful night's sleep or relief in 15 seconds. Who can resist such enticement, especially when the need is very real and immediate? The drugs used in these medications are very potent and often are the same drugs used in the prescription medications, only at a lower strength. The greatest harm done by using these products is the delay that often occurs in seeking professional help. Without an accurate diagnosis from a professional, there is no assurance that the over-the-counter medication selected will be as effective as a prescribed one. Also the relief from the over-the-counter medication is likely to be short-lived because the variety of medications and their strengths can be significantly less than prescribed medications. This reduced duration of effectiveness often means that the patient will take a second dosage of medication prematurely, hoping to obtain the same relief. The patient may experience a more rapid development of tolerance to the drug, resulting in the reduced effectiveness of subsequent dosages and a possible respiratory crisis.

Proper use of over-the-counter (OTC) medications depends on the patient's being informed about the proper way to use medications and the ingredients in them. The patient should consult his physician before taking any medication. Some schools of pharmacy may have an information bureau, which can be an excellent source of information on drug interaction and over-the-counter medications. Patients need to read all the contents listed on the label of an over-the-counter medication. Some of the names for the drugs in the medication may be very difficult to pronounce, but with time the patient will recognize the words and begin to associate them with the desired actions (Table 6-1). The patient should be discouraged from purchasing and using OTC bronchodilator metered-dose inhalers. This type of bronchodilator is easily abused, and the drug used may not have the same effect as a prescribed bronchodilator.

Many over-the-counter cold remedies are combinations of drugs from each of the classes listed in Table 6-1. It is not uncommon for expectorants and antitussive drugs to be in the same elixir. When combined with some prescribed bronchodilators, sympathomimetic drugs may promote the adverse reactions experienced by many patients, even though the sympathomimetic drugs are administered topically. It is not uncommon for combination oral bronchodilators, whether over-the-counter or prescribed, to contain a barbiturate to reduce the adverse reaction to the stimulating sympathomimetics. These barbiturates can have the adverse effect of suppressing the respiratory drive in some patients. Over-the-counter inhaled bronchodilators frequently contain high percentages of alcohol as a diluent. In fact, some of the better-known inhaled bronchodilators contain alcohol that is approximately 64 proof. This alcohol not only has the normal depressant action of alcohol but also tends to dry secretions.

When the patient and her family are being educated about the use of medications,

Table 6-1 Common over-the-counter medications for a cold

Class and ingredient name	Action	Administration	Adverse effects
Sympathomimetics Phenylephrine (Neo-Synephrine) Pseudoephedrine (Sudafed) Phenylpropanolamine (Propadrine)	Decongestant	Topical—sprays Systemic—oral	Increased BP Increased HR Tolerance Taxiphylaxis Necrosis of tissue
Antihistamines Chlorpheniramine Maleate (Chlor-Trimeton) Carbinoxamine (Clistin) Cyclizine HCl (Marezine) Promethazine HCl (Phenergan)	Dry secretions	Systemic	Drowsiness Thickened secretions Decreased clearance of secretions Mucous plugging of airways
Expectorants Potassium iodide (SSKI) Guaifenesin (glyceryl guaiacolate) Ipecac Water (best expectorant)	Increase production and/or mobility of secretions	Systemic	Hypersensitivity reactions Vomiting Nausea May be ineffective
Antitussives Codeine Hydrocodone Dextromethorphan	Suppression of cough reflex	Systemic	Addiction Decreased clearance of secretions Pooling of secretions

it is important that the patient understand the reason she is taking each one. She must also have a clear understanding of the procedures to follow in administering and preserving each medication. The patient should know the side effects of each medication and any possible side effects of combinations of different medications. Special precautions and considerations for operating equipment, driving, or performing other activities should be explained. The best rule to follow for using over-the-counter medications is to take only those medications recommended by a physician. The pharmacology of medications is extremely complex. Information about over-the-counter medications should be communicated to the patient and her family so they may act wisely.

Another class of over-the-counter drugs that could cause a problem for the patient is antihistamines. These drugs can dry secretions, making movement of secretions in the airway more difficult and causing secretions to thicken. These actions can increase the work of breathing, clog airways, and breed infections.

Although a cough can be annoying and a cough suppressant is indicated if the patient is not able to rest, cough suppressants such as dextromethorphan generally are counterproductive. Coughing is a natural and effective means of clearing the lungs of secretions. One cough suppressant, codeine, is like barbiturates because it can depress the drive for respiration and is potentially habit-forming. The action of combined oral and inhaled bronchodilators begins quickly but does not last very long. It is possible to develop a tolerance to these drugs, thus requiring larger or more frequent administrations of the medication to achieve the same effect. These inhaled medications are easily and frequently abused by persons who are uninformed. Also oral and inhaled bronchodilators often contain dosages of theophylline or other drugs that are below the concentration necessary to produce a therapeutic blood level. This low concentration means that the patient is not receiving the greatest benefit from the medication and that potential benefits may not be realized, leading to overuse of the bronchodilator.

IMPORTANCE OF DIET IN A PULMONARY DISORDER

What we eat is important to how we are able to function in life. Ingested foods are metabolized in the cell using the oxygen present to produce energy and build body tissue. Whether we take in the wrong types of foods, not enough food, or too much food, the implications for body function are tremendous. In the pulmonary system poor nutrition leading to semistarvation causes a decrease in vital capacity, minute ventilation, and respiratory efficiency. Without the appropriate amount of glucose, lecithin cannot be produced in a sufficient quantity, and lung function is impaired. Obesity affects the pulmonary system in a restrictive manner, decreasing functional residual capacity and maximal voluntary ventilation and increasing the work of breathing. A deficiency of vitamin A can lead to a loss of ciliated epithelium. And vitamins E and C are needed to aid in protection of the lungs from atmospheric pollutants and oxidative agents.

COMPONENTS OF GOOD NUTRITION AND A BALANCED DIET

Six essential food elements in good nutrition

- Water
- Carbohydrates
- Minerals
- Protein
- Fats
- Vitamins

Components of a balanced daily diet

- Two servings of dairy products per day
- Two servings of protein per day
- Four servings of breads and/or cereals per day
- Four servings of vegetables and/or fruits per day

Much of our dietary behavior is habitual. We eat what we eat and how we eat because we have always done it that way. An extremely important area of life, diet is another part of the rehabilitation of the COPD patient. Modifying eating behaviors is not an easy task, and the problems associated with poor nutrition are multifaceted. The person who is losing or gaining weight despite an appropriate caloric intake should consult a nutritionist. A nutritionist's involvement in a rehabilitation program is a significant asset to patients and the staff.

Educating the patient and his family is the foundation for changing nutritional habits and dealing effectively with the problems the patient may be experiencing. Everyone involved in patient education should keep in mind that education does not change behavior but that the knowledge base must be present for the patient to work toward a change. Many persons are ignorant of the basics of nutrition and a balanced diet. Once these basics are understood, it is helpful to have the patient suggest foods to satisfy nutritional requirements. Personalizing dietary recommendations increases the likelihood that they will be followed after the rehabilitation program. Cultural differences must be taken into account when planning a patient's diet. Some basic information that everyone should know about nutrition is given in the box above. One basic rule of good nutrition is to avoid excess and to eat everything in moderation.

COMMON NUTRITIONAL PROBLEMS OF COPD PATIENTS

Most COPD patients experience similar problems associated with their disorder and nutrition:

Loss of muscle mass or excess weight

Loss of appetite

SOB

Abdominal distension

Tenacious secretions

Dehydration

Electrolyte imbalance (potassium depletion and sodium retention)

Poor general nutrition

Individual needs, which can be identified through the interview and counseling process, should be incorporated into a care plan whenever possible. Once a plan has been established, patient compliance should be monitored, and alterations should be made whenever possible.

IMPLICATIONS OF NUTRITIONAL PROBLEMS

The loss of muscle mass and the carrying of excess weight both have serious consequences for the person with a pulmonary disorder. Each situation can contribute to SOB, weakness, and a decrease in activity levels. These conditions can lead to further deterioration of functional capacity and can contribute to the deconditioning effects of immobility. Weight loss is not usually associated with a loss of muscle mass, that is, protein wasting. It is not clear why some patients with a pulmonary disorder experience protein wasting while others do not. Appearance, specifically body type, is not a clear indication that protein wasting is not a problem. Kwashiorkor and marasmus are both conditions in which protein wasting is present, but the body types in each disorder are very different. In kwashiorkor fluids are retained, swelling the body, and marasmus cachexia is apparent. Protein wasting is an extremely serious condition that must be treated vigorously under the guidance of a physician and a nutritionist.

Loss of appetite has many sources. Medications may be causing nausea, sputum production may be affecting appetite, and SOB may be decreasing motivation to prepare foods as well as eat them. Because of poor nutritional intake, body tissues are not repaired and the ability to fight infection is impaired. In many societies eating is a social function. When a person does not eat, it is difficult to participate fully in these functions. This lack of participation can further isolate the patient with a pulmonary disorder.

SOB at mealtime is perhaps the most common complaint of the COPD patient. It may occur while eating or while preparing a meal. The timing of SOB is important in choosing an approach to solving the problem. SOB at mealtime limits the amount and quality of food eaten and detracts from the enjoyment of eating. The COPD patient cannot enjoy the food or the social atmosphere during a meal when SOB. This lack of enjoyment can contribute to low self-esteem and unwillingness to cope with the disorder.

One mechanism some individuals use to cope with SOB at mealtime is to eat very quickly and to eat only infrequent, large meals. Eating quickly leads to a rapid breathing pattern, further air trapping, an increase in the work of breathing, and more SOB. Air swallowing and subsequent abdominal distension may also increase. This gastric insufflation can contribute to SOB, especially after meals. It can also produce a bloated, uncomfortable feeling and decrease the amount of activity tolerated after a meal. These problems can lead to a fear of eating. The habit of eating three times a day, often with a snack before bed, is partly cultural. The relatively large portions many patients have at these meals can contribute to a feeling of fullness with discomfort and difficulty breathing. Eating frequent, light meals can alleviate this problem.

Excessive sputum production or tenacious secretions also affect the nutritional status of the patient with a pulmonary disorder. Airways become closed or narrowed with mucus, contributing to increased work of breathing and SOB. Thick, tenacious secretions are difficult to remove through coughing or postural drainage, both of which require energy from the patient. Inadequate or inappropriate fluid intake can lead to dehydration, which contributes significantly to the nature of secretions. Secretions that are difficult to remove act as a breeding ground for infection, further sputum production, and deterioration of the patient's condition. Sputum production has been reported to increase after eating spicy foods, but no final explanation can be given for this occurrence.

An electrolyte imbalance can result from inadequate nutrition, but potassium depletion and sodium retention more often are effects of medications. The thiazide diuretics contribute to a loss of potassium. Processed foods and high use of table salt can contribute to an elevated sodium concentration with subsequent fluid retention, edema, and excessive weight gain. Other symptoms that have been attributed to an electrolyte imbalance are muscle weakness, tremors in the extremities, cramps, SOB, and an increased work load on the heart.

Poor nutrition can have many causes, including living alone, low income, physical weakness, poor teeth, and lack of knowledge. The weakness and susceptibility to infectious diseases that result from poor nutrition compound the problem as the patient continues in a downward spiral of deconditioning and worsening symptoms. Misinformation and habits formed over a lifetime are often identified as contributors to poor nutrition and health. The lack of an adequate source for repair of cells and production of energy prevents improvement of symptoms and repair of lung damage.

APPROACHES TO DEALING WITH NUTRITIONAL PROBLEMS

Many approaches to nutritional problems of COPD have been suggested. A creative practitioner with help from a trained nutritionist can identify numerous specific approaches to individual problems. All recommendations must fit into the lifestyle of the patient. If the patient is unwilling to change a specific habit or circumstance, it is her choice, and it will do no good to focus nutritional changes on this area. Some general principles apply to most individuals with a pulmonary disorder. These principles have been found to be helpful in dealing with the implications of nutritional problems. Generally, supplementary feeding and vitamins are not needed for the patient with a pulmonary disorder. This is true as long as the patient's diet consists of foods with a high ratio of nutrients to calories. By reading package labels, the patient can make wise choices when purchasing food.

Training and increased protein intake are required to build muscle mass and to solve the problem of loss of muscle mass. Protein is an expensive element in a balanced diet, so cost must always be considered. Fish, red meat, dairy products, and poultry are all traditionally good sources of protein, but several varieties of beans and legumes can be inexpensive, tasty sources of protein. Adding ¼ cup of nonfat dry milk to foods increases the protein content while not adversely affecting the flavor. The patient with a problem losing weight or the patient who complains of SOB at mealtime will find it helpful to eat a light meal about every 2 hours during the day. Six or more small meals will be tolerated better than three large ones, and snacks composed of high-quality foods should be readily available.

When a patient is overweight, it is important to determine the reason so that the appropriate treatment can be determined. People who are depressed, who have a lifestyle characterized by a low level of energy expenditure, or who have a glandular disorder may be overweight. Eating may be one of the few diversions for the home-bound patient. Professional assistance may be needed to identify the source of the patient's overweight condition and counseling should be instituted when appropriate. Obesity is identified as a gross body weight that is 20% over the calculated ideal body weight. The box below gives the formula for calculating an adult's ideal body weight.

Excessive weight increases the work of breathing and the energy required to perform a given activity. Obesity is associated with increased morbidity in pulmonary disorders and lower FRC. The heart must also work harder to pump blood through an extra ⅔ mile (approximately) of blood vessels for each extra pound of fat. If overeating and lack of activity are the sources of excess weight, a weight-loss diet and exercise are indicated. Basically the key to losing weight is to eat less and exercise more. The overweight person with lung disease should eat a balanced diet that includes small portions from all the essential food groups and exercise regularly. But if the excess weight is from fluid retention, another serious problem exists. A physician must then be consulted, and medications must be adjusted or prescribed.

The source of loss of appetite, such as depression, anxiety, medications, or physical problems, should be clearly identified whenever possible. The loss of appetite may be a symptom of an underlying psychologic or emotional problem that may require professional assistance. Poor dental health may make chewing painful or even impossi-

---

FORMULA FOR CALCULATING IDEAL BODY WEIGHT (IBW)

Male: 106 + (6 × height in inches >5 feet) = lbs.
Female: 105 + (5 × height in inches >5 feet) = lbs.

ble. After a source has been identified, specific recommendations can be made to correct the problem. In general appetite is increased when meals are made as attractive as possible and the setting for the meal is quiet, well-lighted, and comfortable. Eating with friends or other people often helps an individual eat more. If sputum production is a problem, bronchial drainage can be done 1 hour before meals and fluid intake should be maintained throughout the day between meals. Medications that cause nausea can be taken with meals instead of before them, and aerosolized bronchodilators can be inhaled just before eating. Many persons find that light exercise or a small glass of wine before meals stimulates their appetite. Resting for 30 min before meals and not exercising for 1 hour after meals may also be recommended. This will help prevent fatigue while eating and will allow for thorough digestion of food after meals.

SOB during meals is often associated with poor breathing control while eating. By eating more slowly, chewing food well, and pacing swallowing with breathing, that is, swallowing after inhaling and not gulping, SOB can be relieved. Preparing and eating meals requires that energy be expended. By administering oxygen while preparing or eating meals, the increased demand for oxygen can be met. When SOB occurs in association with meal preparation, work-efficiency principles should be applied. This involves preparation of the work space and convenient location of the utensils that are used most often. By preparing casseroles that can be reheated or making "TV dinners" to be reheated, the energy expended and heat generated by cooking can be minimized. The patient should avoid rushing by planning ahead and allowing for a slower pace to avoid taxing herself. Relaxation and elimination of vigorous activity after meals aids in digestion and movement of material out of the stomach, allowing the diaphragm to move more freely. Abdominal distension often leads to SOB. By avoiding gas-forming foods (see the box below), eating slowly to prevent air gulping, and avoiding carbonated beverages, SOB can usually be controlled.

Sputum production during meals often contributes to SOB and loss of appetite. This problem requires forethought to be dealt with effectively. The patient needs to recognize her pattern of sputum production and the length of time after bronchial hygiene and therapy that sputum production is at its lowest. Knowing this allows for planning of bronchial hygiene and meals so that meals can be eaten at times of least sputum production. Tenacious secretions can be controlled with adequate fluid intake. Every person with a pulmonary disorder should drink approximately 30 ml of fluid per

COMMON FOODS AND DRINKS
—— **MENTIONED BY PATIENTS AS CAUSING ABDOMINAL DISTENSION** ——

Cabbage	Broccoli	Nuts	Beer
Beans	Melons	Onions	Radishes
Apples	Sauerkraut	Asparagus	Carbonated beverages

FOODS HIGH IN POTASSIUM

Bananas	Peanuts	Beef	Fresh vegetables
Oranges	Yams	Milk	Prunes
Raisins	Tomatoes	Fish	Beans
Dates	Potatoes	Squash	

---

kilogram of body weight every day. This will add up to 1.5 to 2 quarts or 8 to 10 glasses of fluid per day. The patient's hydration level can be checked regularly by observing skin turgor. Certain fluids, such as alcohol and coffee, should be avoided. These types of fluids do not need to be eliminated, but consumption of them should be limited. Another good rule to follow is for every alcoholic or caffeinated beverage consumed, an equal amount of water should also be consumed. A 2-quart bottle of water in the refrigerator allows the patient to keep track of the quantity of fluid he is consuming. The entire bottle or its equivalent should be consumed every day. In the summer months, during periods of increased sputum production or increased activity, the quantity of fluid taken in should be greater, for example, 2.5 to 3 quarts per day.

An electrolyte imbalance can be quite serious, and symptoms should be closely monitored for patients taking diuretics. For the person experiencing potassium depletion, high-potassium foods should be included in the diet (see the box above). Oral potassium supplements can be prescribed, but the taste of them is unpleasant and not well tolerated and may upset the stomach. Sufficient quantities of potassium can usually be consumed in the diet. The person with edema and fluid retention should choose low-sodium foods, and all cooking should be done without salt. Alternative spices should be used in place of salt. Care should be taken to watch for unusual weight gain or ankle swelling that indicate fluid retention.

A consultation with a dietician is recommended to improve poor general nutrition. Many factors affect a person's lifestyle and eating habits. These factors should be explored thoroughly during an interview, and nutritional alternatives should be suited to the individual's needs. Factors such as dental health and lack of knowledge affect nutritional habits. The patient often needs advice on how to shop for food and how to get the most nutrition for her money. Certain community organizations address the problem of nutrition, especially among the elderly. Such resources should be used whenever possible. Vitamin supplements are only beneficial when the diet is inadequate. If a person is eating properly, additional vitamins are lost in the urine. If a vitamin supplement is recommended, it should contain iron along with the other vitamins and minerals.

The box above suggests some guidelines for daily fluid intake. The patient should always consult her physician before starting a vigorous program of water consumption so that she is aware of any contraindications. Water is the best fluid because it has no

_____ RECOMMENDED INTAKE OF FLUIDS _____

1½ quarts per day for a person without lung disease or with lung disease and a stable, productive cough

2½ quarts per day when fever is present, sputum production increases, exercise is performed, constipation persists, or urine darkens

Alcohol and caffeine, which act as mild diuretics, should be reduced but not necessarily eliminated.

Water is the best fluid. Fruit juices, soft drinks, and milk are allowed, but monitor and limit calories if weight is a problem.

calories and is easily absorbed by the body, but other fluids are also suggested. Moderation (not elimination) of caffeinated and alcoholic fluids is important because of the effects they have on the body. Also there is no evidence that milk increases or thickens sputum production.

When a patient is discharged from the hospital, she may be given a preprinted list of foods as a diet plan. If this list is misplaced or is perceived as confusing or too much of an abrupt change in the patient's lifestyle, it probably never will be implemented. Many varieties of diets (low-salt, low-calorie, low-cholesterol) can be found in bookstores and pharmacies. Although many of these diets are adequate for use by the public, the patient with a pulmonary disorder may require specific counseling, encouragement, and follow-up. Changes in the patient's behavior and attitudes may be essential to treat successfully the nutritional problems of the patient with a pulmonary disorder.

BIBLIOGRAPHY

American Hospital Association: Staff manual for teaching patients about chronic obstructive pulmonary diseases, 1982, The Association.

Christmas Seal League of Southwestern Pennsylvania: Self-help: your strategy for living with COPD, Palo Alto, Calif, 1983, Bull Publishing Co.

Hamilton EM and Whitney E: Nutrition concepts and controversies, pp 55-289, St Paul, Minn, 1979, Western Publishing Co, Inc.

Keys A, editor: In the biology of human starvation, Respiration 1:601, Minneapolis, 1950, University of Minnesota Press.

Moser K et al: Better living and breathing: a manual for patients, St Louis, 1980, The CV Mosby Co.

Petty T et al: Intensive and rehabilitative respiratory care, ed 2, Philadelphia, 1974, Lea & Febiger.

Webber-Jones JE and Bryant MK: Over-the-counter bronchodilators, Nursing 80:34-39, Jan 1980.

CHAPTER 7

Mechanical ventilation, oxygen equipment, and care of equipment in the home

MECHANICAL VENTILATION IN THE HOME

Mechanical ventilation of a patient in the home can have three very important benefits. First, it can improve the quality of life for the ventilator-dependent patient and his family. It can also improve the patient's physical, emotional, and psychologic condition. Second, it can reduce the financial burden of ventilator care on the patient and the community. The costs of home ventilation can be one fourth to one half the cost of mechanical ventilation in an acute-care facility. Third, home ventilation provides an alternative to hospitalization for the ventilator-dependent patient. Most extended-care facilities do not accept ventilator-dependent patients. This means that the only alternative to hospitalization for this patient is a hospice or a home for people with a terminal illness, even though the ventilator-dependent patient is not dying. On the contrary, many years may pass before the patient dies. The patient can still function and contribute to family and possibly to society in significant ways.

A program of mechanical ventilation at home must provide a system of care in the home that meets the medical needs of the patient. Needs should be met in terms of quantity and quality, with the objective of maximizing the patient's functional capacity and potential as a person. Home mechanical ventilation is an efficient use of resources and a practical means of normalizing the lifestyle of many patients.

Assessment of the patient and family

Not everyone who is committed to long-term mechanical ventilation is a candidate for home ventilation. Several conditions for which home mechanical ventilation may be indicated are listed below:

Spinal-cord injury
Neuromuscular disease
Sleep apnea
Obstructive pulmonary disease
Restrictive pulmonary disease
Myocardial and cardiovascular disease
Miscellaneous neurologic diseases or injuries

Yet for many patients in these categories, mechanical ventilation in the home may not be appropriate for a variety of reasons. Three important areas must be evaluated before a program of home mechanical ventilation is implemented. Assessment of each of these areas must include the family as well as the patient. These areas are the emotional, physical, and psychologic aspects of the home environment; the patient; and the family or support network. Stability in these areas greatly increases the chances for success in home mechanical ventilation. An emotionally stable patient and family are able to maintain a good relationship with other people. They do not have a tendency to isolate themselves. Open communication is apparent in the relationships within the family. The patient and family are able to express their thoughts as well as their disappointment, anger, and joy in a nonthreatening way. The psychologic condition of the patient should show a strong desire to live, and family members should demonstrate their desire for the patient to live. The patient on the ventilator wants to be independent and wants to do as much as possible for himself. Physically the patient is stable. No major changes in the patient's ventilatory status are expected, and the likelihood of recovery from the ventilatory disability is poor. These three factors are not easily assessed, so professional assistance should be used whenever possible. An open round-table discussion among all persons involved, including the patient, is an excellent way to assess the situation and to help the family and patient realize what is involved in the commitment to home mechanical ventilation.

Stability and strength in emotional aspects of patient and family relationships should be evident. This stability and strength should be observed in the condition of the patient's marriage and the relationships among family members. Friends and neighbors are welcome in the family's home. Social outlets, for example, through clubs or church, are part of the family's lifestyle. A communication network is available for the patient. Perhaps the patient relates best with his spouse or child. These people can be used as conduits for communication among the people participating in home care.

The patient's medical problems are not the only aspect of physical stability to be considered. There should be no other family members with major disabilities in the home. Obviously two disabled individuals may have difficulty managing each other. Family members must have the strength to move the patient in bed and to move equipment around the room for cleaning. They must also have the stamina to maintain vigilance in monitoring the ventilator. If major psychomotor disability is apparent, it can have a detrimental effect on the outcome of mechanical ventilator use in the home. Many tasks involved in patient care, such as suctioning, require dexterity and good eye-hand coordination.

Having a patient on a mechanical ventilator is a tremendous adjustment for all persons involved. It is imperative that the family have a strong desire to have the patient home. Family members must accept the permanent disruption of the home environment and have the ability to adjust to changes in lifestyle. These are not easy adjustments to make. They require people of at least average intellectual ability with a firm psychologic foundation. A great deal of material must be learned and accommodated over a relatively short period. Mastery of many skills is necessary, but it cannot be accomplished if the participants are unable or unwilling.

Some communities have an abundance of home-care companies that provide home mechanical ventilation, but many have none at all. The availability and capability of health-care providers in these companies is also important (see the section on DMEs, beginning on p. 169). If qualified personnel are not available to provide care, follow-up, and education to the patient and family, home mechanical ventilation should not be attempted. Adequate amounts of the equipment and disposables used in mechanical ventilation must be available to ensure high-quality care. The company also must be able to provide service and backup equipment to the patient if needed. Home-care company personnel, who must be skilled in patient assessment and ventilator management, should visit the family regularly. They should be interested in the details associated with home management of a mechanical ventilator. A positive, constructive attitude on the part of the staff of the home-care company helps the family to provide the best possible care for the patient.

A home-ventilator program cannot succeed without firm support from a physician. As stated in Chapter 1, the relationship among physician, patient, and family remains the key to success in long-term care. A positive attitude toward the home-care program transmitted to the family and the home-care company will encourage high-quality long-term care. The need for extensive nursing care should be minimal. Although it is possible to administer home care to patients with ostomies, special nutritional needs, or complicated medications, these situations make it less likely the family will be able to cope with the entire program.

Assessment of the home environment

Location of the patient in the home is a key factor in providing adequate care and an indicator of the family's willingness to have the patient home. If the room for the ventilator is out of the way, it will not be possible to care for the patient properly or to make the patient an integral part of family life. It is best if the room for the ventilator is in the stream of activity in the home so that every aspect of home life involves the patient. The patient's room must be able to accommodate the patient, the ventilator, and the necessary supplies, as well as the bed or other equipment required to care for the patient. Adequate heating and air conditioning, water for cleaning, and room for storage, drying, and assembly of equipment are important. If the family does not have good housekeeping habits, arrangements may need to be made for an occasional cleaning of the home. Consideration should be given to the size of doorways through which equipment must be moved, the existence and number of stairsteps, and the availability of ramps for the patient to have access to all areas of the home. Finally, adequate telephone facilities should be available both for safety and for maintaining communication between the patient and the physician and the patient and the home-care company.

There must also be adequate electricity available in the patient's room. Grounded outlets are required for medical equipment. The circuit on which the equipment is to be installed should be checked. (See the box below for instructions on mapping electric circuits.)

The total amperage on the circuit must be below the amperage of the circuit breaker or fuse to prevent tripping the breaker or blowing the fuse. Most homes have 15 amp breakers or fuses. The total amperage on a circuit going to a circuit breaker or fuse can be calculated by dividing the total wattage on a circuit by 120. The wattage of an appliance can usually be found on the panel with the information from the manufacturer, such as the model number. This can be important, for example, if a hair dryer is plugged into the same circuit as the ventilator, suction machine, television, room lights, and air conditioner. It is possible to trip the circuit, in which case none of these items will work.

Planning for the discharge of a ventilator-dependent patient

Home mechanical ventilation requires much planning before the patient is ready to be discharged from the acute-care facility. The elements of discharge planning discussed in Chapter 9 should be used as a guide. Generally at least 2 to 3 weeks are required to accomplish all the necessary tasks before the patient can go home. Certainly an assessment of the home and instruction of the patient and family are necessary. Changes to the home may require the services of an electrician or carpenter, and the patient and family may require 20 to 30 hours of instruction before the patient is discharged. The entire home environment, including physical space and the attitudes of persons in the home, will need preparation. The lines of communication among the team providing care and the delineation of responsibilities will require coordination and forethought. If family members see that all aspects of care have been considered,

---

MAPPING ELECTRICAL CIRCUITS IN THE HOME

1. Place a number by each of the circuit breakers or fuses in the main electrical panel.
2. Using one piece of paper for each room in the home, draw a square representing the room and mark each receptacle or light in the room.
3. Make sure each receptacle has a light or small appliance such as a radio plugged into it. Turn on all the lights and radios you have plugged in.
4. Turn off the Number 1 circuit and note the appliances affected (they will be off). Mark the circuit number by the receptacles and lights in that room on the drawing for that room.
5. Turn that circuit back on and turn off the next circuit in the numbering sequence.
6. Continue until all appliances or lights in all rooms have been assigned to a circuit.

TYPES AND BRANDS OF MECHANICAL VENTILATORS

Types of home mechanical ventilators

Time-cycled, volume-limited
Time-cycled, pressure-limited
Chest cuirass, negative pressure
Tank type, negative pressure
Pneumobelt
Rocking beds

Sample of the manufacturers of home or portable mechanical ventilators

Thompson
Life Products
Puritan-Bennett
Emerson
Lifecare
Bourns Bear

---

they will be more comfortable about the program. It is important that the patient and family see the equipment and use it in the hospital before the patient is discharged. This preview allows them to develop confidence in the equipment and demonstrate to the staff their skills in the respiratory-care techniques they have learned. Finally all financial and insurance questions need to be worked out to the satisfaction of all concerned before the patient is discharged.

Features of a home mechanical ventilator

Simplicity in a home mechanical ventilator is essential. Several types and some brand names found in the home are listed in the box above. A ventilator that is simple to operate can make patient care and running and monitoring the ventilator much easier for the family and the company supplying the equipment. Instructions and trouble-shooting methods can be simplified to make them more easily understood by the patient and family. Visual and audio alarms are very important, but they cannot substitute for diligence. Alarms should have different colors and sounds to allow the patient and family to quickly distinguish among the problems that may arise.

Three sources are used to supply power to a portable or home mechanical ventilator: house current, 110 volts AC; an external battery, 12 volts DC automobile battery (operation time approximately 15 to 20 hours); and an internal battery (operation time approximately 1 hour). The batteries can be recharged by the house current, and separate alarms indicate the status of each power source.

The controls on the ventilator may include an on/off switch, a pressure-limit dial and gauge, a low- and high-pressure alarm, the volume setting, a control for inspiratory and expiratory time, a rate control, and sensitivity to inspiratory effort.

Indicators on the ventilator include a delivery-pressure manometer, power source lights and alarms, delivered-volume indicator, visual and audio alarms for pressure, mode, and inspiration, and external low-pressure/disconnect audio alarms.

The circuit to the patient usually consists of standard large- and small-bore tubing with an exhalation valve. A source of humidity, such as a cascade or an artificial nose, is needed. An adaptor for connection of the external low-pressure/disconnect alarm should be available.

At times additional items may be required for home use of the ventilator. Equipment such as a mandatory intermittent ventilation setup will require external gas sources and extra tubing, a reservoir bag, and the appropriate H valving configuration. Any time O_2-enriched inspired gas (Fio_2 >0.21) is required, an external O_2 source is needed. The O_2-enriched gas also requires that gas be blended to achieve the desired Fio_2 and that repeated analysis of inspired gas be made.

The most critical piece of equipment in home mechanical ventilation is the manual resuscitation bag. It must be present at all times in case of ventilator failure. The family needs to be familiar with the assembly, operation, disassembly, and cleaning of the device.

VENTILATOR MONITORING IN THE HOME

Persons working with the ventilator or providing care to the patient must wash their hands before performing any task. The most frequently cited source of infection transmission is the personnel managing the mechanical ventilator or delivering aerosols to the pulmonary patient.

The mechanical ventilator must be checked every 2 to 4 hours, 24 hours per day. There is no time off or holidays from ventilator maintenance. Each check should include examining the circuit-tubing connections, draining water from the tubing (always into a waste container—never back into the humidifier), and maintaining the water level in the humidifier by adding sterile distilled water as needed. Checking the high- and low-pressure alarms requires that someone "bag" the patient during the check. To check the high-pressure alarm, occlude the circuit as the ventilator cycles on and goes to peak pressure. To check the low-pressure alarm, leave the circuit open to the air for a few ventilator cycles and listen for the alarm. Examine the air inlet filter to be sure it is clean. If it is dirty, remove accumulated dust, wash with soap and water, rinse, and replace.

Every one of the regular ventilator checks should be recorded on a ventilator checklist (see Appendix C). The "ventilator checklist" has a place for the date and time of the check and space for recording the present settings on the ventilator controls. The volume set on the ventilator and delivered to the patient, the RR of the ventilator and of the patient, and the system delivery pressure of each delivered breath are important information to be recorded. Other items to be recorded are the pressure-limit setting, inspiratory and expiratory time settings, temperature of inspired gas, inspired O_2 concentration, flow-rate setting, and humidifier setting. External equipment and settings, such as the tank-gauge pressures of the cylinders or O_2 concentrator flow-rate setting and suction-equipment operation, should also be examined. Finally, the individual performing the check should initial the record to show that the task was completed.

If any values obtained during this check are *not* the same as those ordered by the physician, the difference should be noted, and the ordered parameters should be re-established. At times it may be necessary to notify the home-care company or physician. When in doubt, call.

Troubleshooting in the ventilator

Every possible situation that the patient or family may encounter cannot possibly be covered and learned in advance. However, the major problems that are most likely to occur and the corrective action to be taken should be covered (see the box below).

TROUBLESHOOTING GUIDE FOR A HOME VENTILATOR

Low-pressure alarm sounding often or with each breath

- Check all patient connections with the ventilator and the alarms. Look for loose or disconnected tubing.
- Check the cuff on the tracheostomy tube.
- Check for tight connection of humidifier jar.
- Check for water in the tubing to the alarm.
- Check for a leaky or torn exhalation valve.

Decrease in pressure reading during ventilation

- Check all patient connections with the ventilator and the alarms. Look for loose or disconnected tubing.
- Check the cuff on the tracheostomy tube.
- Check for tight connection of humidifier jar.
- Check for water in the tubing to the alarm.
- Check for a leaky or torn exhalation valve.

High-pressure alarm sounding often or with each breath

- Check to see if the patient needs suctioning.
- Check for occlusion of the large-bore tubing, such as with water.
- Check for "crimped" tubing.
- Check tracheostomy tube for occlusion. Clean inner cannula.

Audio alarm at peak pressure

- Battery is running low. Switch to alternate power source.

Complaint from patient of underventilation, SOB, or shallow breath

- Check all of above aspects.
- Remove the patient from ventilator.
- Bag with resuscitation bag.
- Phone for assistance from ventilator supplier.

Ultimately the family and the patient should understand that *when in doubt they should remove the ventilator from the patient and "bag" with a manual resuscitator until help arrives* or until the problem is identified and corrected.

Ventilator maintenance in the home

The patient's breathing circuit should be changed at least every other day. Some circuits are nondisposable and should be cleaned according to the home-care company's instructions. (See the section on equipment cleaning, beginning on p. 131.) Always follow the recommended methods for cleaning a piece of equipment. Some nebulizers, tubes, and other equipment cannot be cleaned and should be discarded after use. In general the entire system should be cleaned at least 3 times per week. Dusting the ventilator daily with a damp cloth prevents dirt buildup in areas where bacteria can grow. Routine ventilator checks should be performed without fail, even when little seems to change. Appendix C contains suggested forms for a ventilator check and an assessment of the patient. Suctioning and airway care should be done regularly when necessary. Too-frequent suctioning and handling of an artificial airway can contribute to trauma and infections.

SYSTEMS FOR THE DELIVERY OF O_2 IN THE HOME

O_2 has been used as a form of medical therapy for more than 100 years, but well-controlled scientific studies on its use have only recently been conducted. Following are some of the benefits of O_2 therapy for the patient with a chronic pulmonary disorder:

Improved tolerance for exercise and activities

Decreased pulmonary hypertension

Decreased erythrocytosis and polycythemia

Reduced mortality and morbidity

Improved neurophysiologic function

Some of the major results of the Nocturnal Oxygen Therapy Trial (NOTT study), an extensive examination of continuous O_2 therapy (18 to 24 hours per day) vs. nocturnal O_2 therapy alone, are listed below:

Patients receiving 12-hour O_2 therapy had 2 times the mortality rate of patients using continuous, 18-24 hour O_2 therapy.

Patients receiving continuous O_2 therapy showed a decreased hematocrit.

Hypoxic pulmonary hypertension was reversed in patients receiving O_2 continuously.

The larger the physiologic derangements from hypoxia, the greater the benefits of continuous O_2 use.

A general conclusion that might be drawn from this study is that continuous O_2 therapy was more beneficial to patients than intermittent O_2 therapy.

O_2 therapy in the home is more common today than it has ever been. Three types of O_2 delivery systems are commonly used in the home: O_2 concentrators, O_2 cylinders, and liquid O_2 reservoirs. Each of these systems has advantages and disadvantages in its operation and application. The type of system to use for a specific patient is a decision that is best made by examining the lifestyle and rehabilitation goals of the patient. In general the more aggressive the plan for self-care and active the patient's lifestyle, the more mobile and convenient the O_2 system should be.

The O_2 concentration in the lungs of a patient receiving O_2 therapy is a function of the type of equipment used, the flow rate of the gas, and the rate and depth of patient ventilation. To determine whether a patient is receiving a sufficient amount of O_2, the volume of O_2 in the blood must be measured. This can be done by either invasive or noninvasive means, such as an ABG assay or pulse oximetry.

O_2 CONCENTRATOR

An O_2 concentrator is a device developed using "space-age" technology. The basic principle of operation is separation of the 21% O_2 from the 78.8% nitrogen (N_2) in the atmosphere. The O_2 is then compressed and stored in a small cylinder for use by the patient. The outside of the equipment can be attractive. It may even have the appearance of a piece of furniture, such as an end table. It can be moved from room to room on wheels and can operate on the 110-volt household electrical current. Some are able to use the 12-volt electrical current found in automobiles. O_2 concentrators are simple to operate and maintain. An on/off switch is all that is needed to operate the machine, and there are few user-serviceable parts. There is no requirement for refilling as there is with cylinders, and an annual overhaul is usually all that is needed for continued operation. For a patient requiring continuous long-term, low-flow O_2, an O_2 concentrator can be the most cost-effective of the O_2-delivery systems available.

There are some disadvantages to the use of an O_2 concentrator. Some O_2 concentrators produce a constant rumble or hum, as well as heat. Because the concentrator is powered by electricity, an increase in the electric bill can be expected. The concentrator must be located close enough to an adequate electrical system, so new circuits or more modern wiring may be needed in some locations. If a power failure were to occur, an alarm would notify the patient that the concentrator is not operating, and a backup O_2 system, usually a cylinder, would be necessary. The concentrator and backup system take up floor space, which could be a problem in a small apartment. Even though it is somewhat mobile, the concentrator cannot be considered portable. For exercise or activity outside the home and for travel and business, a separate O_2 system will be needed. For a patient who is not homebound, the need for a separate system can be a major disadvantage.

Operation of the O_2 concentrator

Each brand and model of O_2 concentrator has unique characteristics, but the principles of operation are not extremely different. Once the O_2 has been extracted and compressed into a near 100% concentration, the O_2 therapy is not too different, from a patient's point of view, from any other O_2 therapy equipment. The most commonly used method of separating O_2 and N_2 is the N_2-absorbing sieve bed. A second method, the semipermeable membrane, can also be used to produce O_2 from air. This method does not produce concentrations of O_2 near 100%. Generally the gas produced is between 35% and 50% O_2, depending on the flow rate to the patient, but it is 100% humidified.

A simple explanation of the process of N_2 absorption through the sieve beds follows. Filtered air is drawn into the nitrogen-absorbing sieve bed by a vacuum generated by the compressor. As the air moves through the sieve bed, nitrogen is absorbed by sodium aluminum silicate crystals. The gas that exits from the sieves is dry, very high in O_2, and very low in N_2. This gas is routed to a small internal cylinder for storage. As the patient uses the O_2, it is drawn from the cylinder, and the contents of the cylinder are replenished. This process is continuous. Two sieve beds are usually needed. One bed absorbs N_2, and the other bed is purged of the nitrogen accumulated in the chemicals. This purging is done by drawing some of the near 100% O_2 through the sieve bed. The N_2 purged from the sieve bed is expelled into the atmosphere (Fig. 7-1). Because small amounts of air are involved in the extraction process and because the rooms and homes in which the machine is used are open, the patient can be assured that there is no danger of depleting the O_2 from the room in which the concentrator is located. The extraction process in an O_2 concentrator is *not* perfect; therefore the concentration of O_2 produced is nearly 100% (>95%). The concentration of the O_2 produced is primarily dependent on the flow rate of the gas to the patient. As the flow rate at which the gas is delivered increases, less time is allowed for N_2 absorption, so a lower "purity" of O_2 is compressed in the storage cylinder. Some concentrators can produce <97% O_2 at a low flow rate (1 to 2 L/min). Medical-grade O_2 cylinders, hospital-piped gas systems, and home liquid O_2 systems always deliver O_2 at a concentration of >99% purity. This difference between the concentration of O_2 from a concentrator and the gas concentration from other systems has no practical implications for the patient receiving O_2 therapy at low flow rates. For higher flow rates (>3 to 4 L/min) the characteristic inefficiency of N_2 absorption of each concentra-

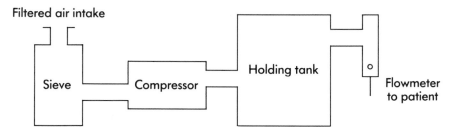

Fig. 7-1 Internal diagram of the nitrogen-absorbing O_2 concentrator.

tor must be considered. A flow rate of 5 L/min may be needed from a concentrator to achieve the same Pao_2 in a patient that can be had at 3 L/min from another O_2 system.

Considerations in the decision to use an O_2 concentrator

An O_2 concentrator is an excellent choice as the means for delivering O_2 to a patient when the need is long-term and the flow rates must be low (<4 L/min). An O_2 concentrator is an appropriate means of O_2 delivery when the patient's condition limits physical activity outside the home and when the physician's prescription includes the following conditions:

Flow range of 1 to 4 L/min at rest or with activity

Continuous use of O_2 therapy (18 hours per day or greater)

O_2 delivered through a low-flow device, such as a cannula

Patient's ADL limited to home

If the conditions appear to be closer to those seen in the list below, then another O_2 delivery system may be more economical and may better meet the needs of the patient.

O_2 needed only during exercise or activity

Prescribed flow-rate range greater than 4 L/min

Intermittent use or use less than 18 hours per day

Aerosol therapy prescribed with O_2

O_2 therapy through high-flow O_2 device

Inadequate electrical wiring, no ground

Inadequate amperage on electrical circuit

When the need for O_2 is intermittent (occasionally during the day or sporadically for brief periods of time), a concentrator is not the appropriate O_2 therapy device. It is also inappropriate if the patient is ambulatory, occasionally goes outside the home, or does not have access to an adequate source of electrical power.

Important points on use of an O_2 concentrator

The utility company supplying electrical power to a patient's home should be notified that an O_2 concentrator is being used in the home so that in the event of a power outage, the home with the concentrator will receive high priority to have electrical power restored. This notification and gaining of priority may require explaining what a concentrator is and why the utility company should care. A thorough check of the total amperage on the electrical circuit with the concentrator will prevent overloading the electrical supply. In general the total amperage should not exceed 15 amps. In many homes an electrical hazard may exist if 15 amps on a circuit is exceeded (see the box on p. 117). Only a three-prong, grounded electrical outlet should be used with the concentrator. Receptacle "cheaters," or two-prong adapters, should not be used to bypass the medical-grade electrical plug on the concentrator.

O$_2$ CYLINDER

The major advantages of using O$_2$ cylinders in the home are the relatively low cost and the well-established technology. Cylinders are quiet when they are delivering O$_2$, and the patient can be assured of receiving 99% O$_2$ at all times, even at high flow rates. Cylinders are used in all parts of the world for O$_2$ delivery. A patient can be assured that O$_2$ cylinders will be available almost anywhere in the United States the patient may travel. The technology of compressed gas in a metal cylinder and of the regulators and flowmeters is more than 100 years old. Considerable progress has been made to standardize cylinder sizes, fittings, and connections throughout the country.

There are some disadvantages to using cylinders for O$_2$ delivery. The cylinders are bulky (a large cylinder weighs approximately 150 pounds, and a smaller cylinder weighs approximately 25 pounds). The cylinder is under extremely high pressure, approximately 2000 pounds per square inch gauge (psig); the working pressure of the equipment is 50 psig. Use of cylinders for O$_2$ delivery in the home means that cylinders will also be needed outside the home for activities such as walking or shopping. A member of the patient's family must have the mechanical ability and strength to change regulators and transfill small cylinders from the large ones for ambulation.

Each size of cylinder has a limited capacity that dictates how long it can operate at the needed flow rate. Its duration is measured in hours and minutes of gas flow. The limited capacity of a cylinder requires frequent replacement of cylinders in the home and refilling of portable cylinders for use outside the home. A cylinder should never be emptied completely. Some pressure, called a "heel," is left in each cylinder, and the cylinder is considered empty when the heel is reached. In small cylinders, such as sizes D and E, a heel of 500 psig is used. Large cylinders, such as sizes M, G, and H, may use a heel of 200 psig. The purpose of the heel is to prevent atmospheric humidity from entering the cylinder and damaging its internal walls. The heel can also provide a margin of safety so that the patient will not be without some O$_2$. The calculation of tank factors, the duration of cylinder operation, and the use of the heel are given in the boxes on p. 126. The patient and/or the family must be comfortable in performing these calculations (see Appendix H).

Considerations in the use of O$_2$ cylinders

In theory, O$_2$ cylinders can be used whenever and wherever O$_2$ therapy is needed. But there are some problems with using them. Cylinders can be impractical in some physical settings, such as a small apartment, and with prescribed flow rates over 3 to 4 L/min. They may also be impractical for many patients because use of cylinder O$_2$ can conflict with a patient's lifestyle and with the goals of the patient's rehabilitation program. For example, if a physician wants a patient to exercise regularly and the patient must wear O$_2$ to do it, the number of cylinders used could be very high. If the patient is active and enjoys activities such as shopping, going to the theater, and

CALCULATION OF TANK-USE FACTORS,
L/PSIG, AND CYLINDER DURATION OF OPERATION*

$$\text{Tank-use factor} = \frac{\text{cu/ft full} \times 28.3 \text{ L/cu/ft}}{\text{psig full (2200)}}$$

Example: Tank factor for an H cylinder of O_2:

$$\text{Tank-use factor} = \frac{244 \text{ cu/ft} \times 28.3 \text{ L/cu/ft}}{2200 \text{ psig}} = \frac{6905 \text{ L}}{2200 \text{ psig}} = 3.14 \text{ L/psig}$$

Tank-use factors for cylinder sizes

	D	E	
L/psig	0.18	0.28	
Number of L from full to 500 psig	306	482	
Number of L remaining at 500 psig	90	140	
	M	G	H or K
L/psig	1.57	2.38	3.14
Number of L from full to 200 psig	3139	4854	6302
Number of L remaining at 200 psig	314	476	628

*The capacities and duration of full O_2 cylinders are given in Appendix H.

CALCULATION OF
THE DURATION OF A CYLINDER AT ANY GAUGE PRESSURE

$$\text{Duration in minutes} = \frac{(\text{Tank pressure} - \text{Heel}) \times \text{Tank factor}}{\text{delivery flow rate}}$$

Example: A K cylinder with 800 psig pressure operating at 2 L/min:

$$\frac{(800 \text{ psig} - 200 \text{ psig}) \times 3.14 \text{ L/psig}}{2 \text{ L/min}} = \frac{1884 \text{ L}}{2 \text{ L/min}} = 942 \text{ min}$$

$$\frac{942 \text{ min}}{60 \text{ min/hour}} = 15.7 \text{ hours}$$

$$(60 \text{ min/hour} \times 0.7 \text{ hours}) = 42 \text{ min}$$

Answer: 15 hours, 42 min

visiting, a portable cylinder may not last long enough for the patient to complete the planned activity. A liquid system would allow an active patient to continue to function in a manner as near normal as possible. If the need for O_2 is intermittent and short-term and low flow rates are required, then an O_2 cylinder is usually the system of choice. The box on p. 127 contains some guidelines to consider when deciding whether to use O_2 cylinders for a patient.

SITUATIONS TO CONSIDER BEFORE DECIDING TO USE O₂ CYLINDERS

Situations in which O₂ cylinders may be appropriate

O₂ flow rates of 1 to 2 L/min for a few hours per day

Short-term, intermittent need for O₂

    Only at night while sleeping

    Only with exertion or ambulation

Whenever the usage rate would not equal the cost for an O₂ concentrator

Wherever an O₂ concentrator is indicated but available electrical circuits are inadequate to support the concentrator

High-flow O₂ therapy, Venturi masks, and aerosol devices requiring 100% O₂ or a 50 psig source gas

Situations in which O₂ cylinders may be inappropriate

Long-term, continuous, low-flow O₂ therapy

O₂ flow rates of 2 to >4 L/min for ≥18 hours per day

When frequent visits to replace cylinders would be impractical or economically inappropriate because of geographic location

When the patient is active and away from home for long periods (approximately 4 hours or more)

PRECAUTIONS FOR USE OF O₂ CYLINDERS

1. Cylinders must be secured to the wall by a chain or bar or to the floor by a cylinder stand.
2. O₂ cylinders must be stored in a dry, cool, well-ventilated area, not in a closet.
3. The patient should not move large cylinders once they have been secured by the supplier.
4. All cylinders should be kept at least 10 feet from heat sources, such as sunlight, heating ducts, radiators, and electrical motors.
5. A large cylinder should never be moved with the regulator attached.
6. The parts of a cylinder or regulator should never be lubricated.
7. Cylinders should be moved only when in the cylinder cart.
8. The cylinder should not be carried by the valve stem or regulator.
9. A cylinder should never be emptied completely. It should be changed when the heel is reached.
10. The local fire department should be notified that O₂ is being used in the home.

Guidelines for O₂ cylinder care in the home

The care, cleaning, and maintenance of O₂ therapy equipment is not complicated. The surfaces of the equipment should be kept clean and free of dust and dirt. The equipment should not be used for any purpose other than the intended one. For example, a regulator should not be used as a hammer, and a cylinder should not be used as a coat rack. There are some rules to follow for using O_2 equipment in the home. These rules were developed for the safety of the patient and family and for the care of the equipment. Some of the more important safety measures and rules to be observed when using O_2 are listed in the box on p. 127. These rules, developed by the National Fire Prevention Association (NFPA) and the Compressed Gas Association (CGA), apply whenever O_2 is in use.

LIQUID O_2 RESERVOIR

A liquid or cryogenic O_2 system has a number of advantages over either of the other two systems for O_2 delivery that have been discussed. With a liquid O_2 system, a large quantity of O_2 can be stored in a very small space. For example, a container for liquid O_2 the size of an end table can hold O_2 equivalent to 5 or more large K cylinders. The liquid O_2 is delivered to the patient's home in a reservoir and is measured by pounds as opposed to the liters and cubic feet of a cylinder. Reservoirs come in a variety of sizes: 20-, 30-, and even 50-pound capacity. A typical patient receiving O_2 at 2 L/min may need a 30-pound reservoir, which could be sufficient for 1 month. This same patient would require 14 to 16 K cylinders of O_2 each month. The convenience of the small reservoir becomes apparent when the inconvenience of having 16 large cylinders in the home is considered. This inconvenience does not even take into account the ambulatory difficulty experienced when cylinders are used. The amount of O_2 a patient would need for a 1-month period and the cost-effectiveness of the liquid system can be calculated (see the box below). However, it is important to note that the calculation of cost-effectiveness for any O_2 system does not take into account the patient's lifestyle, rehabilitation goals, or capacity for productive activity. If the patient

---

DURATION OF OPERATION FOR A LIQUID RESERVOIR O_2 SYSTEM

Given: 1 lb liquid O_2 = 0.14 cu/ft liquid O_2
          Liquid O_2 expands 860 times to a gas; units of measure are the same
          1 cu/ft gas = 28.3 L gas

Example: (2 L/min O_2 × 1440 min/day) × 30 days/mo = 86,400 L/mo

(0.14 × 860 × 28.3) = 3407.3 L/lb.

$$\frac{86,400}{3407.3} = \sim 25.4 \text{ lb/mo}$$

26 pounds liquid O_2 = 3.64 cu/ft liquid O_2 = 3130 cu/ft gaseous O_2 = 88,579 L gaseous O_2

88,579 L divided by 6215 usable liters of gas = 14.2 K cylinders O_2

(Total cylinder capacity − Heel = Usable liters)

is very active, the liquid system may be most appropriate, even though the flow rate prescribed may indicate otherwise.

A liquid O_2 reservoir is similar to a large Thermos bottle. Whether large or small, the reservoir insulates the liquid O_2 and maintains a proper low temperature until needed. As the patient uses O_2, some of the liquid is converted into its gaseous state by passing through a warming coil. The gaseous O_2 is stored in a small cylinder to be delivered to the patient through a flowmeter at the prescribed flow rate. The entire system operates at a relatively low pressure, 50 psig, and produces no noise. A small, portable, liquid cylinder can be filled from the main reservoir. When it is full, it will weigh about 5 lb. This portable liquid reservoir can hold enough O_2 to allow the patient to be away from the main reservoir for up to 8 hours. This portability and convenience permits the patient to maintain a lifestyle as near normal as possible and to remain active in many activities. Some patients continue to work and enjoy other activities that would not be possible with any other system for O_2 delivery.

There are some disadvantages to the liquid O_2 system. The gas exists in the reservoir as a super-cold liquid gas (approximately $-280°$ C). This has the potential to cause a "cold" burn if the liquid O_2 is handled improperly. The risk of "cold" burn is greater for the personnel delivering the gas than for the patient. The large reservoir for the liquid O_2 has a connection for filling the portable cylinder. This connection can become very cold after the filling procedure and should not be touched. A liquid O_2 system may be more expensive than the other systems because of the cost of the technology and the cost of the liquid O_2. The reservoirs for the liquid O_2 are not perfect insulators from the warm temperature of a room relative to the temperature of the liquid O_2. A small amount of O_2 is lost to the atmosphere. The amount that is lost can be minimized by training the patient and the family to use the portable reservoir as prescribed and not to overfill it.

ADVANCES IN HOME O_2 ADMINISTRATION

Recently there has been emphasis on conserving the O_2 being delivered to patients. An attempt is made to achieve the same Pao_2 in a more efficient manner. A lower flow rate of O_2 is delivered to the patient; therefore less O_2 is used, and the monthly cost is reduced. The traditional O_2 prescription assumes a continuous flow of O_2 to the patient. During inspiration, O_2 is added to the room air being breathed, raising the fractional concentration of inspired O_2 (Fio_2). When the patient exhales, the O_2 is still flowing to the patient, so all the gas during this phase of respiration is blown into the room. Some conserving devices use reservoirs to capture the wasted gas and allow it to be breathed again. Other devices use advanced technology to achieve a similar end. The basic equipment used to administer the O_2 therapy to the patient, such as a cannula or mask, is essentially the same as in traditional O_2 therapy. Modifications to improve efficiency are made to the flow-metering equipment or to storage systems.

The Oxymizer pendant or Oxymizer moustache are examples of devices using a reservoir to better control the O_2 used by the patient. These devices look like a large cannula. The pendant model has a round "bag" reservoir that rests below the chin on the chest, and the moustache model has an elongated reservoir located under the nose. The gas flowing to the patient during exhalation is captured in the reservoir to be inhaled on the next breath instead of being blown out into the room. A lower O_2 flow rate than would be required with a traditional cannula can be used to achieve the desired level of O_2 in the arterial blood.

Another method of reducing the amount of O_2 needed to maintain an appropriate Pao_2 uses a microcomputer chip and a selenoid valve to start the flow of O_2 during inhalation and stop it during exhalation. The chip senses the beginning of inhalation and opens the valve, allowing a bolus of O_2 to be delivered to the patient. Three mechanisms for conserving O_2 have been developed using this technology.

The first method is the detection of inspiration by a flow sensor. When inspiration is detected, a precise amount of O_2, for example, 16.5 ml, is delivered at the beginning of inspiration. This bolus of O_2 at inspiration has the equivalent effect of a flow rate of 1 L/min. A 33 ml bolus is equivalent to 2 L/min. A second method uses slightly different technology to sense the negative pressure generated at the nose at the beginning of inhalation. A selenoid valve is opened that allows a continuous flow of O_2 at a high rate until the end of inhalation is sensed and flow is stopped. The third mechanism is similar to the other two. It delivers a precise amount of O_2, such as 35 ml, at different times in the ventilatory cycle. Each of these devices can be added to a standard O_2 cylinder or liquid O_2 system to reduce the amount of gas needed by the patient.

The conservation devices mentioned above use standard respiratory-therapy equipment for O_2 delivery to the patient. Gas flow to the patient is controlled to make its use more efficient. Transtracheal O_2 therapy uses the standard storage methods for O_2, cylinders, and liquid but administers the gas directly into the trachea instead of into the nose. The original idea for this method of delivery was developed several years ago. A cardiac catheter placed through the neck into the trachea was used to deliver O_2 to patients with COPD and heart disease. The patients were able to use a lower flow rate of O_2 to maintain their Pao_2 at the same level as with traditional O_2 therapy methods. Modifications to the cardiac catheter have since been made, and catheters designed for transtracheal O_2 therapy, such as the SCOOP system, are now available.

Although catheterization is an efficient method of O_2 delivery, it is not the best choice for every patient needing O_2. It is an invasive procedure during which the catheter is placed into the trachea through a permanent opening in the neck. Before this procedure is prescribed, the patient should require long-term O_2 therapy and be prepared to undergo surgery. Though the stoma in the neck for the catheter can close after the catheter is removed, catheterization should not be considered a temporary method of O_2 therapy.

Patients using transtracheal O_2 therapy report better compliance with O_2 therapy, especially in public. The O_2 tubing can be threaded under the patient's shirt and connected to the catheter. The catheter is hidden by a high collar or ascot, and persons around the patient may not be aware that the patient is using O_2. The improved compliance and the lower flow rate of O_2 are key benefits of this method of O_2 therapy.

CARE AND CLEANING OF RESPIRATORY-THERAPY EQUIPMENT IN THE HOME

Bacteria on respiratory equipment can be a major source of respiratory infection for the patient with a pulmonary disorder. If a nebulizer is contaminated with bacteria, the aerosols produced deposit bacteria in the respiratory tract along with the medication. Such contamination makes nebulizers a major source of respiratory-tract infection, perhaps second only in disease transmission to poor hand washing.

Thoroughly cleaning and disinfecting or sterilizing equipment can stop contaminated equipment from causing pulmonary infection. The steps for cleaning and disinfecting respiratory equipment are outlined in the box below. Cleaning is defined as the

---

STEPS IN CLEANING AND DISINFECTING EQUIPMENT

Disassemble equipment as completely as possible.
Wash in mild, nonperfumed detergent.
Rinse with hot water.
Soak in solution of acetic acid for 20 to 30 minutes (one part white household vinegar, one part distilled water).
  Mix only enough disinfecting solution to submerge the equipment. Discard solution at least every 5 to 7 days.
  Keep solution in the refrigerator, covered, between uses.
Rinse in hot water.
Allow to air dry. Do not blow with hair dryer.
Cover with a towel to prevent dust from settling on equipment while it is drying.
When dry, store equipment in a sealed plastic bag. Mark the date the equipment was cleaned on the bag.

1:1 ratio of vinegar to distilled water = 2.5% acetic acid
1:3 ratio of vinegar to distilled water = 1.25% acetic acid

Alternatives
1. Bleach solution: soak in a 1:10 solution of bleach to distilled water. Rinse in a 1:3 solution of acetic acid and water. Then rinse in water and air dry before use.
2. Boiling for 15 minutes to disinfect (near sterilization).

Always: Allow equipment to air dry while covered with a cloth.
         Package with as little handling as possible.
         Date all equipment and solutions.

removal of sputum, dirt, and particulate contaminates from a piece of equipment. Cleaning with soap and water is the best way to remove these materials. Disinfection suppresses bacteria growth on a piece of equipment but does not kill all the bacteria or destroy all the spores.

A solution of 2.5% acetic acid has been shown to be an effective and inexpensive disinfectant. This solution can be made at home by mixing 1 part white household vinegar, which is approximately 5% acetic acid, with 1 part distilled water. For patients who find the odor of acetic acid in a room or on equipment intolerable, a weaker solution can be mixed, but disinfecting with acetic acid requires a minimum concentration of 1.25%. This low concentration can be obtained by mixing 1 part vinegar and 3 parts distilled water. A bleach solution, consisting of 1 part chlorine bleach and 10 parts distilled water, can also be used to disinfect equipment. It is especially important that equipment disinfected with a bleach solution be rinsed thoroughly before use. It may be necessary to soak the equipment in an acetic-acid solution (mixed as described above) after submersion in the bleach solution to aid in removing the bleach before the equipment is used.

Sterility is the absence of all life forms on the equipment and is the best condition under which to use equipment. Working in sterile conditions is difficult to do with the majority of equipment used in home care. Boiling equipment for 15 minutes is the closest way to sterilize it, but most equipment will not tolerate boiling. Heating towels and other equipment in a partially open oven at approximately 250° F for 15 minutes can disinfect this type of material. Only equipment that can tolerate the high temperatures of boiling or the oven should be sterilized in this manner, and caution should be used when placing material in the oven.

The respiratory-therapy department in many hospitals provides equipment-sterilization services to patients. Several times each year, usually at least every 6 months, a patient can bring in all equipment and for a fee have it sterilized using ethylene oxide. Having equipment sterilized professionally is a good practice because organisms are not killed by disinfection and are thus allowed to grow.

How to clean and disinfect equipment

Disinfection can be economically and reliably performed to reduce the occurrence of aerosol-transmitted infection. Respiratory-therapy equipment used several times in a day should be rinsed after each use in water, shaken to remove excess water, and covered until the next treatment. A daily routine of cleaning and disinfecting should be rigidly followed (see box on p. 133). It may be necessary to have more than one set of equipment, such as two or three micronebulizers. This would allow the equipment in use to be rotated. For example, one nebulizer can be used while the other is being disinfected. Any item that is designated as disposable should be discarded when indicated and not kept for later use. Frequently, disposable equipment is not designed for complete disassembly; therefore it cannot be cleaned and disinfected properly.

ROUTINE FOR
CLEANING AND DISINFECTING RESPIRATORY EQUIPMENT

Daily

Clean and disinfect small reservoir nebulizers.
Discard unused portion of reservoir water.
Refill humidifiers with distilled water.
Check the cannula or mask for dirt. Discard if necessary.
Dust surfaces with damp cloth.

Weekly

Clean and disinfect all equipment at least three times a week.
Replace mask, cannula, and O_2 connecting tubing.
Check filters for cleanliness.

Following are some general rules to follow when cleaning and disinfecting equipment and when using supplies:

Never leave any equipment uncovered or unpackaged.

Never skip cleaning and disinfecting.

Never reuse disposable equipment after it should be discarded.

Date all solutions.

Date all packaged disinfected equipment.

Never use solutions that are past the expiration date or discolored.

Never use solutions with questionable contents.

Making solutions for respiratory care

A great deal of distilled water and saline is used in therapy administration and equipment cleaning in pulmonary home care. The patient can save money by preparing at home some of the solutions for use in therapy. Sterile distilled water can be produced by boiling distilled water for approximately 15 minutes. The distilled water can be purchased from the grocery store or obtained by running tap water through a filter attached to the faucet. The filter should be of sufficient quality to remove bacteria and chemicals from the water. The filter should be changed regularly to maintain optimum function.

The inside walls of any container holding a sterile solution or used to produce a sterile solution should never be touched. Sterile water can be prepared by placing a clean glass container into a pot of tap water (Fig. 7-2). Fill the inside container with distilled water and bring the water in each container to a boil. After boiling the water for 15 minutes, turn off the heat, cover the pot and the container, and allow them to cool. When the water has cooled, cap the container, remove it from the pot, and mark

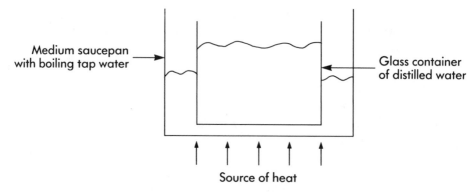

Fig. 7-2 Setup for preparation of sterile water at home.

the date and time on the jar. Store the jar of sterile distilled water in the refrigerator with the refrigerated medications. Use only the amount of sterile water necessary for each treatment. Pour the needed volume into a small container. If too much is poured out, discard it. Never return the unused portion to the container from which it came. All sterile water should be discarded after 5 days even if it appears safe to use. With time the patient will learn the volume of solution to mix for a 5-day period of therapy, and waste will be reduced.

Normal saline can be produced at home by mixing *¼ teaspoon noniodized salt into 1 cup sterile distilled water.* Larger quantities can be made by increasing the amounts in the formula, for example, by mixing ½ teaspoon of salt into a pint of water or a full teaspoon of salt into a quart of water. Remember to date all solutions and to discard unused portions after 5 days.

BIBLIOGRAPHY

Bell W et al: Home care and rehabilitation in respiratory medicine, Philadelphia, 1984, JB Lippincott Co.

Christopher KL et al: Transtracheal oxygen therapy for refractory hypoxemia, JAMA 256:494-497, 1986.

Fischer DA and Prentice WS: Feasibility of home care for certain respiratory-dependent restrictive or obstructive lung disease patients, Chest 82:739-743, 1982.

Fleig CP: Double quats: disinfectant alternative to vinegar, Rx Home Care, June 1982.

George RB: Mechanical breathing devices for use at home, Am Lung Assoc Bull 7-11, Dec/Jan 1978.

Gilmartin M and Barry M: Home care of the ventilatory dependent person, Respir Care 28(11):1490, 1983.

Hodgkins JE, Zorn E, and Connors G: Pulmonary rehabilitation: guidelines to success, Stoneham, Mass, 1984, Butterworth Publishers.

Hunter PM et al: Home mechanical ventilation manual, 1984, Publishers Glasrock Home Health Care, Atlanta, Ga.

Krop HD, Block AJ, and Cohen E: Neuropsychologic effects of continuous oxygen therapy in chronic obstructive pulmonary disease, Chest 64(3), 1973.

Lilker ES, Karnick A, and Lerner L: Portable oxygen in chronic obstructive lung disease with hypoxemia and cor pulmonale, Chest 68(2):236-241, 1975.

Make B et al: Rehabilitation of ventilator-dependent subjects with lung diseases: the concept and initial experience, Chest 86(3):358-365, 1984.

McCue P: Benefits of transtracheal oxygen therapy, Resp Mgt 18(2):23-28, 1988.

Moser K et al: Shortness of breath: a guideline to better breathing, ed 3, St Louis, 1983, The CV Mosby Co.

Neff TA: Selection of patients for oxygen therapy, Chest 68(4):481-482, 1975 (editorial).

Nocturnal Oxygen Therapy Trial Group: Continuous or nocturnal oxygen therapy in hypoxemic chronic obstructive lung disease: a clinical trial, Ann Intern Med 93:391-398, 1980.

O'Donohue W: Mechanical ventilation in the home, sponsored by The American College of Chest Physicians, Travenol Laboratories, Inc.

O'Ryan JA and Burns DG: Pulmonary rehabilitation: from hospital to home, Chicago, 1984, Year Book Medical Publishers, Inc.

Pennsylvania Society for Respiratory Therapy, Inc: Respiratory home care procedure manual, 1983, Philadelphia, Pa, The Society.

Petty TL: Prescribing home oxygen for COPD, 1982, Thieme-Stratton Publishers, Inc.

Petty T et al: Intensive and rehabilitative respiratory care, ed 2, Philadelphia, 1974, Lea & Febiger.

Rozenberg T: Home care: cleaning of equipment, Respir Ther 67-70, May/June 1973.

Schwartz JS et al: Air travel hypoxemia with chronic obstructive pulmonary disease, Ann Intern Med 100:473, 1984.

Sivak ED, Cordasco EM, and Gipson WT: Pulmonary mechanical ventilation in the home: a reasonable and less expensive alternative, Respir Care 28(1):42-49, 1983.

US Department of Health and Human Services: Guidelines for the prevention and control of nosocomial infections, 1982, Public Health Service, U.S. Centers for Disease Control.

Wenmark WH: Suggested guidelines for respiratory therapy home care, (revised 1978), Dallas, Tex, American Association for Respiratory Care: Committee on Rehabilitation and Continuing Care.

CHAPTER 8

Performing respiratory care
in the home

HOME RESPIRATORY CARE

Respiratory therapy is often associated with the application of some piece of medical equipment to aid in the relief of symptoms. Although such equipment can aid in the delivery of medications and the application of therapeutic treatments, supplying it for home use should not be considered a final step in the relief of symptoms or the treatment of a pulmonary disorder. Judicious use is enhanced through instruction and supervision by a trained health-care practitioner to ensure safety and effectiveness. Adequately administering many therapeutic modalities requires cooperation from the person receiving the therapy. A good general rule to follow in the use of respiratory equipment in the home is the simpler it is, the better patient compliance and cost-effectiveness will be.

AEROSOL THERAPY

Patients with obstructive pulmonary disorders often receive an aerosol treatment of a bronchodilator or a "bland" solution, such as saline, at some time during treatment. Aerosols are defined as particles suspended in a gaseous medium. The objective of inhaling these droplets into the lungs is to relieve symptoms such as bronchospasm and tenacious secretions.

Administration of an aerosol in the acute-care setting is supervised by a respiratory-care practitioner. In the home the person receiving therapy must take responsibility for administering treatment in the best possible manner. Learning the proper procedure for administering an aerosol treatment is a major focus in the education of the patient and family. A relatively small amount of the aerosol produced by a nebulizer is actually deposited on the airway (some sources report less than 10% of the total volume nebulized). For this reason it is important that administration techniques maximize the amount of aerosol deposited in the lungs. One feature of a micro-nebulizer that can enhance the inhalation of aerosols is a "thumb control." A small opening, a T piece, or a hole in the O_2 tube just before the nebulizer allows for control of nebulization. The patient can cover the hole or T piece with a finger at the beginning of inhalation and remove the finger at the beginning of exhalation. The medication is nebulized during inhalation only, preventing the medication from being blown into the room during exhalation. Although controlling nebulization increases the time required to administer treatment, more of the medication gets to the patient's lungs, where it is needed.

Administration of an aerosol treatment

The physician's complete prescription should be reviewed with the patient receiving therapy and anyone else who may be assisting the patient. Frequency of administration, duration of the treatment session, and the name and dosage of the medication to be used must be very familiar to everyone involved in patient therapy. Thorough instruction and practice at disassembly and reassembly of the aerosol generator, such as a small reservoir nebulizer, is also important. The patient should be able to name the various parts of the device and be skilled at troubleshooting. The box below gives suggestions for administering an effective aerosol treatment to a patient. The material is divided into procedures to be done before and during a treatment that can improve deposition of aerosol in the lungs and add to the efficiency of the treatment.

ADMINISTRATION OF A MICRONEBULIZER TREATMENT

Before the treatment

Check all equipment to be sure it is clean and dry.
Assemble the nebulizer and connect it to the nebulizer tubing.
Put the correct dose of medication in the nebulizer.
Turn on the compressor or other pressurized gas source.
Cover the "thumb" control to observe the production of mist from the mouthpiece of the nebulizer.

During the treatment

The patient should sit upright, support the back, and relax. Sitting in a semireclining position with a pillow under the knees will relax the abdomen.
Breathe normally with the nebulizer connected to the gas source and the gas source turned on.
Place the nebulizer mouthpiece, which can act as a tongue depressor, into the mouth.
After a normal exhalation and the end of a tidal ventilation (FRC), cover the thumb control to begin nebulizing the medication.
Inhale slowly and deeply until the lungs are full of air. Release the thumb control to stop nebulization.
Pause for 3 seconds, holding breath and aerosols in the lungs.
Exhale slowly and passively to the normal ending point of exhalation. Use pursed lips to exhale if indicated.
Cover the thumb control again. Inhale slowly and deeply until the lungs are full of air. Release the thumb control to stop nebulization.
Exhale slowly, passively, to the normal point of exhalation.
Pause occasionally to take several regular breaths without the nebulizer turned on to prevent hyperventilation.
Repeat the breathing pattern for inhalation of all the medication.

Continued.

┌───┐
│ ──────── **ADMINISTRATION OF A MICRONEBULIZER TREATMENT**—cont'd ──────── │
│   │
│ **Suggestions for a more effective treatment**   │
│   │
│ Use of a thumb control on the nebulizer allows for coordination of medication │
│   nebulization with inspiration. This coordination prevents medication from being │
│   wasted by keeping aerosols from being generated and then blown into the room │
│   during exhalation.   │
│ If the patient cannot coordinate nebulization with inspiration using the thumb control, │
│   an aerosol reservoir can be placed between the nebulizer and the patient to collect │
│   aerosol particles.   │
│ The nebulizer should be held in the upright position throughout the treatment. │
│ The mouthpiece should be placed well into the mouth to act as a tongue depressor. │
│ The lips should be sealed around the mouthpiece. A nose clip may be needed to ensure │
│   inhalation through the mouth.   │
│ When using an MDI without a reservoir or spacer, see the discussion of MDIs on p. │
│   139.   │
│ Monitor HR during therapy. Take pulse at the beginning, in the middle, and at the end │
│   of the treatment.   │
│ With an increase in HR of >20 beats/min from the beginning, *stop*.   │
│ With onset of dizziness or "tingles," *stop*, check HR, rest, and then continue only when │
│   feeling better.   │
│ Notify the physician if not feeling better after a rest or not returning to the beginning │
│   HR.   │
│ A nebulizer treatment requires about 15 minutes to complete. It should be continued │
│   until all medication is nebulized.   │
│   │
└───┘

Equipment for aerosol therapy

Three types of nebulizers are commonly used in administration of aerosol therapy: the hand-held micronebulizer, which has a small reservoir; the entrainment nebulizer, which has a large reservoir; and the ultrasonic nebulizer (USN). A vast array of pneumatic nebulizers are on the market today, and each operates in essentially the same way, no matter what brand is used. The USN is electronically powered and has a much greater output than a pneumatic nebulizer.

A nebulizer with a small reservoir is used for short treatments (10 to 15 minutes long). Treatments are typically for administering a bronchodilator or other medication to the lungs. A nebulizer with a large reservoir is used to administer longer treatments (≥30 minutes) or to apply aerosols continuously, as in a bypassed upper airway (tracheostomy). A bland aerosol, such as sterile distilled water, is usually administered in this manner. The USN is electronically powered and produces a high-density, high-volume output. The USN's output can be adjusted to as much as 10 ml/min. The other nebulizers produce about 2 to 3 ml/min. Particles from the USN are very small and are uniform in size, allowing a great deal of aerosol to be placed into the smaller airways. Bland aerosols are used in the USN but usually only for intermittent therapeutic treatments 15 to 20 minutes in length.

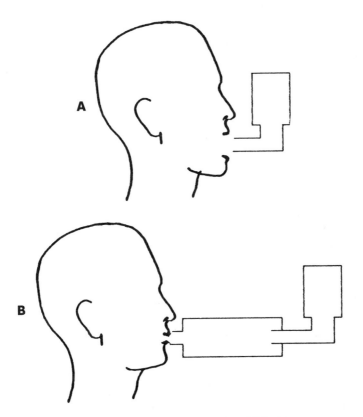

Fig. 8-1 A, MDI without spacer. **B,** MDI with spacer.

The MDI has become an effective, convenient, and therefore popular means of administering aerosols to the airways. It is lightweight and works quickly (a treatment can be over in a matter of 2 or 3 minutes). Each dose from the device is precisely measured and is consistent for each application. Approximately 200 breaths of medication can be received from a typical MDI. The usual medication in the device is a bronchodilator, but steroids and steroidlike drugs are also available in MDIs. Coordination of the breath with triggering of the canister to release the medication can be difficult for some people. Reservoirs are available to aid in the delivery of the aerosol (Fig. 8-1). Because a drop in temperature causes the pressure in the canister to drop, making the MDI less effective, the MDI should be warmed before it is used when the weather is cold. This can be done by keeping the MDI in the hand in a pants pocket or under the arm or by rubbing it vigorously for several minutes.

Several points are particularly important when using an MDI. An MDI mouthpiece can be cleaned in the same manner in which other nebulizers are cleaned, and the canister of medication should not be boiled. When inhaling from the MDI, the patient should not close the lips completely around the mouthpiece of the device unless a reservoir (spacer) is being used. By holding the device near the lips with the tongue down and the mouth open wide, air can be entrained, along with the aerosol generated, to carry the particles deep into the lungs. Inhalation should be slow and deep and should be held for 3 seconds and then followed by slow, passive exhalation. The patient should wait 1 minute before inhaling a second dosage, if prescribed. This pause allows the first inhaled aerosols to deposit and act on the airways so that the next MDI breath hopefully will deposit aerosols even more deeply into the lungs. Because of their convenience, MDIs can be abused by patients. It should be emphasized that like any medication, the MDI should be used only as prescribed. If relief of the wheezing or SOB is not obtained after inhaling the prescribed dosage, the physician should be notified.

IPPB as a means of administering aerosol therapy plays little if any role in home respiratory care. Although it has been used as a method of aerosol delivery, it is not economical and is inappropriate for treatment of obstructive pulmonary disorders. IPPB does have some value in treatment of restrictive disorders or neuromuscular disorders, in which underventilation is a major problem. It can assist the patient to take deeper breaths, facilitate a cough, prevent alveolar hypoventilation, or enhance deposition of an aerosolized medication. Thorough training in the administration of this type of respiratory treatment is required. Particular attention should be paid to the hazards of its use.

The use of impellor-type aerosol-producing room humidifiers should be avoided. These devices are extremely difficult to disinfect and have been identified as a source of respiratory infection. If low humidity makes breathing uncomfortable, the patient should first increase the amount of water ingested during the day. Humidifiers that produce only vapor and no aerosols can add some moisture to a closed room but are generally ineffective in increasing the humidity in a house with many open areas.

BRONCHIAL HYGIENE

In the normal lung approximately 100 ml of mucus is produced every day. In the lower airways the secretions are thin and watery, moving toward the mouth primarily through the action of the cilia that line the airways. As the secretions approach the trachea, the mucus thickens. Normal ADL can enhance the movement of secretions in the airways through the disrhythmic ventilation patterns that occur during activity.

Patients with excessive secretions in the airways may have a mucus-production level 3 to 5 times that of a normal person. Some of this increase is the result of overproduction of mucus by mucus-producing glands that have hypertrophied and by an edematous epithelium. Much of the mucus results from an increase in the number of mucus-producing goblet cells as a response to the chronic irritation in the airway. A normal ratio of ciliated epithelium to goblet cells is approximately 5:1. In bronchitis this ratio may reach 3:1.

Overproduction of mucus affects the lungs and gas exchange in several ways. Airways that do not allow free air movement can contribute to underventilated alveoli, increased levels of $Paco_2$, and lower levels of Pao_2. WOB is elevated as airway resistance increases. Alveolar collapse may result from chronic underventilation. In addition, the pooling of these excessive secretions can provide an opportunity for bacteria growth. Finally, airways filled with thick secretions and narrowed by inflammation and edema contribute to dyspnea and limited functional capacity.

Postural drainage

This therapeutic modality requires the positioning of a patient so that the airway to be drained is in its most vertical position. This way, gravity is able to facilitate the movement of secretions out of the airway. The adult lung has approximately 23 generations or branchings of the airways. This makes positioning complicated. It is often impractical for timely treatment and patient tolerance to attempt to drain off each of these airway branches. However, it is possible to drain the segmental and lobar branchings in the lungs, which creates a possibility of 12 to 18 positions in a full regimen of postural drainage. In acute care the full range of 12 to 18 positions every 2 to 4 hours may be indicated. For the patient at home, four to six positions performed in a prophylactic manner twice each day are usually sufficient to maintain the patency of the airways. Any program of postural drainage must be accompanied by a routine of adequate hydration. It may take a week of adequate fluid intake, approximately 30 ml/kg/day, before the secretions become noticeably thinner. The effectiveness of the postural drainage therapy is lessened when it is not accompanied by adequate fluid intake.

There are two clear indications for postural drainage: to prevent the accumulation of secretions and to mobilize retained secretions. Prophylactic postural drainage is appropriate in these three general situations:

A history of increased sputum production

Prolonged bed rest

Splinting from pain and hypoventilation

The situation that is most pertinent to rehabilitation and continuing care is that of the person with a history of increased sputum production. Prevention of airway closure from mucus accumulation is the primary objective in the use of postural drainage for the person with chronic bronchitis, cystic fibrosis, or bronchiectasis. Patients confined to prolonged bed rest, such as paralyzed patients or patients using home mechanical ventilation, also benefit from prophylactic therapy. A second indication for postural drainage is the retention of secretions, over several days or weeks, in the airways (see the box on p. 142). This accumulation of secretions may subsequently affect the function of the lungs and thorax.

Many of the contraindications to various bronchial-hygiene techniques occur only in the hospital setting. The signs and symptoms listed in the box on p. 142 are typical

---
MOBILIZATION OF RETAINED SECRETIONS

Preoperative or postoperative secretion control
Drainage of a lung abscess
Documented pneumonias and atelectasis
Neurologic disorders or drug overdose

CONTRAINDICATIONS FOR POSTURAL DRAINAGE

Possible contraindications

Pneumothorax
Pulmonary emboli
Hemoptysis
Bullous emphysema
Orthostatic hypotension
Recent surgery (<48 hours earlier)
Abdominal or thoracic aortic aneurysms
Cerebral vascular disorders
Esophageal anastomosis
Complaints of:
    Sharp pain in the chest
    Sudden onset of SOB
    Pink sputum (may be caused by some inhaled medications)
    Dark-brown sputum (indicates presence of old blood)
    Bright-red sputum (indicates presence of new blood)
    Ankle swelling or a significant (3 to 5 pound), sudden weight gain

Definite contraindications

Untreated tension pneumothorax
Hemoptysis that is active or of unknown origin
Unstable cardiovascular system
The period immediately following surgery
Pulmonary edema associated with congestive heart failure (CHF)
Uncorrected aortic or abdominal aneurysms

---

of many disorders. They are complaints often associated with disorders requiring postural drainage. Recognition of these signs and symptoms should act as a warning that postural-drainage therapy is needed. In all these situations the contraindications to the therapy must be weighed against the hazards of retained secretions before continuing the therapy. When this question arises, patients should consult their physician.

As with most therapy the personality of the patient will alter the effectiveness of bronchial hygiene. A patient who is nervous or impatient often finds it tedious to maintain positions for the required amounts of time. Compliance from these patients is often poor. Because therapy is needed on a routine basis, it is often necessary to change the patient's lifestyle. Older patients often find it difficult to move and change positions for the therapy. This makes performing some postural-drainage positions extremely difficult if not impossible.

Following are some patient conditions and situations in which caution would be required when performing postural drainage:

Nervous patients upset with the inconvenience of therapy

Elderly patients (Brittle bones and poor mobility can make some positions difficult.)

Patients with poor systemic circulation and possible emboli

Patients who have recently had surgery on the spine, neck, or back

Discomfort or intolerance in some postural-drainage positions may be due to physiologic disorders. For example, O_2 desaturation can occur in the head-down position because of increased ventilation-perfusion mismatch. A complaint of SOB by the patient should be investigated thoroughly, and steps, such as O_2 administration, should be taken to correct the problem when possible. For patients with poor systemic circulation the possibility of thrombi forming and emboli circulating should be considered. Patients who have had back surgery should not perform positions in which the risk of injury is great or the alignment of vertebrae cannot be ensured. Close monitoring during therapy can minimize risk to the patient.

The two basic components of bronchial hygiene are (1) postural drainage with or without percussion and vibration and (2) various coughing techniques. In the acute-care facility the person experiencing excessive secretions may need postural drainage as often as every 2 hours using eight or more positions. In the home a modification of this in-patient program of postural drainage is necessary to improve compliance while maintaining the effectiveness of the therapy. Generally the patient at home who maintains each of the following positions for 10 to 15 minutes will be performing effective therapy:

Supine—feet elevated 18 inches

On right side—feet elevated 18 inches

On left side—feet elevated 18 inches

Prone—feet elevated 18 inches

Additional positions are listed in Appendix E. Prescribed positions should be kept as simple as possible to facilitate compliance with the therapy.

If specific lung lobes or segments are involved, such as in bronchiectasis and cystic fibrosis, the particular position for that area should be used. It is best to perform this therapy at least twice a day, for example, in the morning and before retiring at night. The patient should hold each position for no less than 10 minutes. Some positions will be tolerated better than others, and the patient's intolerance to a position may necessitate spending less time in that position. The total time for each therapy session should be 45 to 60 minutes. For example, holding four positions for 10 minutes each would equal 40 minutes total time. More frequent sessions, for example, three or four per day, may be indicated when an infection is present or increased mucus production is noted. Routine postural drainage increases the effectiveness of the cough and helps to maintain the patency of airways.

When preparing for postural drainage, the patient should consider the timing of therapy in relation to other activities. Therapy should be performed 1½ to 2 hours after a meal and not too soon before a meal. Coordination of therapy with the administration of medications and other treatments and exercises is also important. In general, waiting 20 minutes after taking a medication, such as a bronchodilator, allows the medication adequate time to take effect. When using a bland aerosol, it is best to perform postural drainage immediately after the aerosol treatment.

Vibration and percussion, the application of mechanical energy to the chest wall with the intention of dislodging and moving retained secretions from within the airways, may be incorporated into postural-drainage therapy. These techniques have been found to increase expectoration of secretions. Mechanical vibrators/percussors are available to help the patient and/or family members to perform the procedures. However, manual vibration can be learned easily and is more economical. Vibration is performed by placing the hands on the patient's chest and applying firm pressure with a rapid shaking motion against the chest wall during exhalation only. Percussion is accomplished by gently striking the patient's chest wall over the desired lung area with cupped hands in a rhythmic fashion. These techniques can be performed alternately for 2 to 4 minutes each while performing each position during a postural-drainage session. A frequency of 10 to 15 vibration or percussion cycles per second has been reported to be the ideal number of repetitions for the mechanical movement of secretions in the airways, but this frequency is achieved only by using mechanical vibrators and percussors.

Percussion is performed by cupping each hand (fingers and thumb together with the palm of the hand curved), creating an air cushion between the hand and the chest wall. The person performing the percussion should keep her shoulders, elbows, and wrists relaxed and flexible. The hands should strike the patient's chest wall rhythmically with equal force at a consistent rhythm and rate (approximately two strikes per second). Extreme force should be avoided. Vibration of the chest wall and the underlying airways is accomplished by placing both hands on the chest wall over the area to be vibrated. The patient should take a very deep breath. During exhalation, slight pressure is applied to the chest, and the arms and hands of the one performing the vibration on the patient are shaken vigorously. Percussion or vibration should not be performed on bare skin. The patient's chest should be covered with a shirt or towel before these techniques are administered. It is not necessary to perform both percussion and vibration during each session of postural drainage. Each procedure can be used alone, giving some relief to the person performing the procedure on the patient. A mechanical vibrator/percussor is believed to be more effective than manual methods because the energy can be applied equally over the chest for longer periods of time at higher frequencies. Vibration and percussion should be performed over the lung area only. Breast tissue and the bony areas of the chest, such as the spine, scapula, and sternum, should be avoided. If the patient has a history of rib fractures or has a skin rash on the chest, these procedures should not be used.

Techniques to improve the effectiveness of a cough

An effective cough is an essential component of proper bronchial hygiene and should be included as part of most respiratory therapy. The cough seems like a simple maneuver, requiring little effort or forethought, but for the person with a pulmonary disorder an effective cough may seem impossible. Many people have had chest colds, in which tenacious secretions have "lodged in the back of the throat" and could not be expectorated easily, creating a very uncomfortable feeling. This is how many patients with pulmonary disorders live all the time. These patients must be trained to perform an effective cough, using the pulmonary capacity they have to expectorate secretions and open airways.

There are several steps to producing a normal cough. First, inhale deeply, using the diaphragm and other accessory breathing muscles. Follow this by closing the glottis and contracting the muscles of the chest and abdomen. This contraction generates a high intrathoracic pressure, approximately 200 cm H_2O or more. Next, open the glottis and rapidly expel the air. The flow rate achieved at this point is likely to exceed 300 L/min. Any secretions located in the trachea will be blown out of the airways into the laryngeal pharynx, where they can be swallowed or expectorated.

There are some very important points about the production of an effective cough. A cough is most effective at high lung volumes (vital capacity) and at high expiratory flow rates. A vital capacity of 20 ml/kg is considered minimal for a cough. Some persons with pulmonary disorders have a reduced vital capacity and cannot achieve appropriate flow rates during exhalation, rendering their cough ineffective. The cough removes secretions from the trachea and possibly either of the two main bronchi. Secretions in the lower airways may be moved toward the mouth during the cough, but even a "deep cough" does not bring up secretions from the periphery of the lungs. The function of the mucociliary escalators and the characteristics of the secretions also influence the effectiveness of the cough.

The importance to effective coughing of conditioning the airways with adequate hydration, postural drainage, and possibly the use of bronchodilators cannot be overstated. An effective cough can be produced in any of three ways: (1) the forceful exhalation or "normal" cough, (2) the staccato cough, and (3) the huffing cough. The forceful exhalation is explosive and usually consists of one forceful effort followed by inhalation. It is tolerated and performed satisfactorily by persons who have normal lung function, that is, those who can achieve high volumes and high flow rates. During forceful exhalation, intrathoracic blood pressure and airway pressure and intracranial blood pressure can be extremely high. This may not be the most efficient method of clearing the airway of secretions, but most people never consider an alternative because normal coughing works quite well for them.

The staccato cough requires less energy than a forceful exhalation and is quite effective in removing secretions from the airway. It is basically exhalation in steps after one deep inhalation. Two or three coughs are produced from the same breath. The first cough has the most force, and subsequent coughs facilitate movement of the secretion out of the airway. It is like a "clearing of the throat" cough, but the staccato cough is done with greater force. The repeated closure of the glottis required for this cough can be taught by pronouncing "K," "K," "K" during a forceful exhalation. The staccato cough is an effective, efficient means of clearing the airway that requires less energy than the "normal" cough. This efficiency can be especially important for patients with bronchitis or other disorders with large amounts of sticky, tenacious secretions requiring frequent coughing. The staccato cough can also reduce the trauma experienced by the vocal cords in coughing.

A third type of cough, the "huffing" cough, involves deep inhalation with incomplete closure of the glottis during forceful exhalation or no closure at all. The technique can be learned by pronouncing the word "hufffff." The "Hu" of the "huff" sound keeps the glottis from completely closing and prevents buildup of large intrathoracic pressures. The deleterious effects of these pressures on the heart, the great vessels of the thorax, and the transmission to the intracranial vessels are minimized, especially in the highly compliant lung with emphysema. The "fff" at end exhalation provides some expiratory resistance, which, like pursed-lip breathing, can prevent early airway closure and air trapping. The huffing cough may be slightly less effective compared with the other coughs. It reduces the trauma of the cough and can be performed by patients who cannot generate the high intrathoracic pressures needed in the other coughing maneuvers.

Some additional techniques that can increase the effectiveness of a cough are serial coughing in increasing intensities, hyperinflation, mechanical coughing, and the "quad" cough. The increasing intensity of serial coughing is performed in the following manner: Inhale a small volume of air and cough when exhaling it. Next, inhale a larger volume of air and cough when exhaling it, then inhale as large a volume as possible and cough vigorously during exhalation for the most effective of the coughs. This coughing technique allows the patient to become used to coughing, especially if the patient experiences pain when coughing. Serial coughing allows the patient to gain confidence in her ability to control the cough and any discomfort it may bring, that is, to splint the site of pain. In addition, any secretions in the airways are moved up from the smaller airways to a position for expectoration.

For the patient who is tracheostomized or intubated, the hyperinflation mechanical cough can facilitate removal of secretions. This coughing maneuver requires the use of a manual resuscitator to hyperinflate the lung and to act as a closed glottis by allowing intrathoracic pressure to build during exhalation. The patient's lungs are inflated with the manual resuscitator. After an inspiratory pause, the patient contracts the abdominal and thoracic muscles, or the health-care practitioner carefully exerts upward pressure on the patient's abdomen. Both of these actions build intrathoracic pressure as the gas in the thorax is compressed against the closed valve in the manual resuscitator. At this point the resuscitator valve is opened, and the release of pressure is allowed to drive the secretions in the airways out. The patient should always be ventilated between efforts to maintain adequate oxygenation and alveolar ventilation.

For the patient who is quadriplegic or whose cough mechanism is suppressed because of paralysis of a portion of the chest, the quad cough can be used to clear the airway. "Quad-coughing" requires a second person to push on the patient's upper abdomen. This pushing should be inward and upward toward the diaphragm. It should be applied during exhalation only and must be coordinated with the efforts of the patient. Compression of the lateral aspect of the chest can also be effective, especially if the patient is lying on the side. Because of the tremendous energy required to push effectively on the patient's abdomen and the discomfort that a person with an intact nervous system can sense, this technique should not be performed on patients who are not quadriplegic.

The position of the patient while coughing can alter the effectiveness of coughing. It is best that the patient sit up and lean slightly forward when coughing. If the patient is required to remain prone, a slight head-down position, semi-Trendelenburg, is helpful. Support should be applied during coughing to the abdomen and to any incisions. A pillow on the abdomen or on the site of pain and gentle pressure applied to this area during the cough minimizes any discomfort. Splinting of the abdomen during a cough can increase the effectiveness of the cough. This is especially true for patients with flaccid abdominal muscles because the patient is able to "work" against the splint to increase the force behind the cough. Patients who have just had upper abdominal surgery can reduce discomfort from coughing by splinting the site of the incision during a cough.

Frequently a forceful cough is followed quickly by an inhalation, which can trigger another cough, setting off a "coughing jag." A "rest breath" should follow a cough; that is, the patient should inhale through the nose and exhale through pursed-lips before making a second effort at coughing. When this rest breath is placed between coughing attempts, the cough can be controlled and the deleterious effects of the cough minimized. Uncontrolled coughing should be avoided because it can lead to syncope, dyspnea, and high intracranial and intrathoracic blood pressure.

Assessment of home respiratory care

An assessment of the bronchial-hygiene program should be done routinely. The person performing the therapy needs to be trained to recognize the components of effective therapy and to know when to suspect a problem or a need for change. The easiest and best measure of the effectiveness of therapy is daily sputum production. An attempt should be made to evaluate the volume, color, consistency, and odor of the sputum produced during each therapeutic session and for several hours later. Any changes in symptoms, such as an increase in SOB or a decrease in exercise tolerance, may be indications of an exacerbation of the pulmonary disorder, requiring an increase in the frequency or intensity of bronchial-hygiene techniques. A daily diary or record of symptoms is a good means of keeping track of the character of the pulmonary disorder and the effect of therapy. The patient's ability to breathe deeply and cough without performing postural drainage and the absence over several days of a productive cough may indicate that the frequency of therapy can be decreased. The decision to alter therapy should be done only in consultation with a health-care professional familiar with the patient's disorder and symptoms.

ENERGY CONSERVATION IN ADL

As described in Chapter 5, patients with chronic disabilities frequently fall into a downward spiral of inactivity. Because the patient becomes uncomfortable, for example, experiencing SOB, when performing certain activities, the tendency is to avoid those activities. This inactivity in turn can cause deterioration of the unused muscles and bones. As the patient adapts to the new level of inactivity, she finds that she is able to do even less than before. It is important that SOB or fear not be allowed to limit unnecessarily the patient's level of functioning.

There are a number of ways to make tasks easier or more tolerable. An occupational therapist (OT) is trained to help people maximize their potential within the limits of any handicaps, making an OT an asset to the health-care team. The OT can train patients and make specific suggestions for overcoming problems they may be experiencing.

Many suggestions for making a task easier seem to be common sense. Because each person without a disability has so much reserve energy for ADL, the need for efficiency is not recognized. The box on p. 149 lists several suggestions for making tasks less stressful and for conserving energy while performing them. In general, unnecessary motion should be minimized, and the patient should avoid rushing through activities. Planning allows the patient to set up the proper conditions for any activity.

The body has a limited amount of energy, which is used up relatively quickly, so a patient should allow for frequent rest periods throughout the day and especially during activities to replenish the supply of energy. Heavy chores should be done during the period of the day when the patient seems to have the most energy. For example, many people feel best and strongest at the beginning of the day, but others don't "get going" until later in the day.

Activities calling for lifting, reaching, pulling, or pushing should be performed while exhaling slowly through pursed lips. If the activity is to be performed over a prolonged period, such as cutting the lawn or pushing a shopping cart, it is important to pace the activity. The patient must avoid holding the breath (Valsalva's maneuver) during any exertion. This maneuver can increase transpulmonary pressure and de-

**SUGGESTIONS FOR ENERGY CONSERVATION
AND STRESS REDUCTION DURING ACTIVITIES**

Minimize steps by planning ahead.

Use tools, such as wheeled carts or electrical devices, whenever possible to help complete activities.

Arrange work area to reduce reaching and bending.

Sit whenever possible and use good posture.

Breathe properly when performing an activity (for example, coordinate exhalation with exertion).

Schedule regular rest periods, such as 10 min/hour.

Work at a slow, comfortable pace, avoiding jerky motions.

Establish priorities. Avoid developing urgent needs.

Spread heavy and light tasks throughout the day.

Maintain an uncluttered work area. Organize utensils and tools according to their use.

Keep work area at a proper height, standing or sitting: just below the elbow (usually 30 to 32 inches high).

crease the amount of blood returning to the heart and the brain. For example, when lifting an object from the floor, the patient should bend the knees, not bend from the hips, and exhale while lifting the object.

Activities such as walking or stair climbing are part of everyday life for most people. Both are also excellent exercise activities for the person with a chronic pulmonary disorder. But these activities also can be strenuous and may provoke fear in the patient. During stair climbing the patient should monitor the pace and coordinate breathing with climbing. Inhaling for one or two steps and exhaling for three or four steps helps to maintain the 1:2 ratio learned from the VREs in Chapter 4. The patient should rest at the end of each exhalation and on the landings. Climbing the stairs in this manner takes a longer time, but the patient arrives at the top of the stairs experiencing much less SOB. With practice and training, it is possible to build endurance to a point at which little or no rest is required and the patient is able to climb stairs almost as well as people the same age. Walking during ADL should be paced to the patient's breathing pattern, for example, inhale while taking two steps and exhale while taking four steps. The RR should be maintained at a normal level, <20 breaths per minute. The patient should avoid holding the breath and should rest whenever needed. Walking can be an excellent exercise, and the more walking that is done, the better the patient will tolerate it (see Chapter 5). Other suggestions for promoting efficiency in several activities of personal care are listed in the box on p. 150.

Climate can have a major effect on the breathing and comfort of the patient with a chronic pulmonary disorder. If the air is cold, the patient should wear a mask and be sure to inhale through the nose. The patient should stay out of wind and walk slowly.

ENERGY CONSERVATION DURING PERSONAL CARE

Bathing

Use a stool in the tub or shower to sit whenever possible.
Use a long-handled scrub brush to avoid excessive reaching.
Use an extension hose in the shower to direct the spray.
Turn on cold water before hot to reduce steam.
Rest periodically.
Use O_2 at dosage prescribed for exercise.
Avoid strong-scented soaps and shampoos.

Grooming

Sit whenever possible.
Rest periodically.
Support elbows on the table, sink, or counter top.
Coordinate motion of combing hair, shaving, or putting on makeup with breathing.
  Exhale during exertion.
Avoid using aerosols or strong scents.

Dressing

Plan ahead. Gather all clothes together before starting.
Wear loose-fitting, easily put on, comfortable clothing.
Coordinate breathing with motion, for example, exhale while bending and inhale while
  reaching.
Slow the pace of activity.
Rest periodically.
Use suspenders in place of a belt.
Put on more than one item at a time, such as underwear and pants or skirt. Avoid
  unnecessary motions.

Most people are comfortable when the relative humidity is between 30 and 50%. An evaporation (pass-over) type of humidifier adds moisture, and a dehumidifier takes it away. Cleaning the humidifier is important, and fresh, new water should be added daily. In warm weather the patient should increase fluid intake and wear light clothing.

Other good rules for the patient to follow are to avoid people who have colds or other communicable illnesses, learn to recognize conditions that trigger breathing problems and avoid them, get adequate rest at night and allow for rest during the day, exercise regularly, eat a balanced diet, and stay in communication with the physician.

RECORD KEEPING AS AN AID IN SELF-CARE

The patient with a pulmonary disorder should keep a record of daily activities, symptoms, and problems complying with the home-care program. This record is an invaluable asset to the health-care worker outside the home who is helping the patient.

With this information the patient can be assisted to recognize activities or situations that can be avoided, thereby preventing some of the discomfort of the disability. A daily diary of symptoms, which characterizes the patient's disabilities, is an aid to the physician when prescribing medications, recognizing problem situations, and counseling the patient. The best program for continuity of care is individualized to meet the needs of the patient. A daily record of symptoms kept over several months that notes the time of day when a symptom occurs and attempts to gauge the severity of the symptom is a tremendous tool in education and treatment. Appendix C includes samples of some charts for the patient's record keeping. These charts include a record for daily symptoms, a record for exercise, and a chart for ADL.

Use of the symptoms chart can probably be discontinued after a few months unless the patient has an exacerbation of the pulmonary disorder or simply wants to continue. These charts should be shared with the physician, and a copy should be kept in the patient's file in the physician's office. By also saving these charts at home, the patient can compare present symptoms with symptoms experienced in the past. Decisions about whether symptoms have improved or worsened can then be made based on some objective data. When telephoning the physician's office with a question or concern, other health-care personnel involved with the patient's treatment can already be familiar with the characteristics of the patient's condition and improve patient treatment. Some training may be needed to ensure the data collected by the patient or family is of good quality. Because it results in better communication and health care, time spent educating and training the patient and family is time well spent.

The exercise record initially should be kept simple and should include only the exercises and activities that have been prescribed for the patient. As the patient's condition improves or the patient becomes bored with the exercises originally recommended, new exercises can be added. The example in Appendix G can be overwhelming to a patient who has just been discharged from the hospital but would not be inappropriate for someone who has been involved in a care program for several months. Compliance with the program can be improved by keeping the chart simple and by regular follow-up by the physician. By recording in the blocks provided the number of times the exercise is performed and/or the amount of weight lifted, the progress of the patient can be assessed. As strength and endurance improve, it will be necessary to increase the intensity of the activity or add new exercises requiring greater energy expenditure. If building strength and endurance is not a goal but the patient simply needs to remain mobile and active, then variety is very important. A number of exercise alternatives are shown in Appendix G. (See Chapters 5 and 6 for more information on exercise training.)

During a program of training in rehabilitation activities and self-care, a record of the patient's ADL will be needed. This record allows the health-care staff to counsel the patient on changes in lifestyle that may be needed. It is likely that the patient with the disability will need suggestions on therapeutic treatments, scheduling exercise as part of a daily routine, and other aspects of the program. By keeping an hourly record of daily activities over several weeks, the patient can recognize the lifestyle patterns that have developed. The patient's usual time of rising and retiring, opportunities for rest during the day, the time of day when the patient's energy level is highest, and ADL that can be used as part of an exercise program should be noted. In cooperation with the health-care team, the patient should develop a daily schedule that includes all the various activities in the care program and the patient's ADL. If this schedule is developed during the care program, when there are opportunities for frequent counseling, adjustments can be made to accommodate the lifestyle of the patient and the demands of the program. The patient should try to follow the schedule for several days and then discuss any problems with the health-care team. It will probably become apparent quickly that the patient's former lifestyle will need to be adjusted to allow adequate time for the new care program. It is best if this is the conclusion of the patient and not a demand by the physician or the program staff. In time the patient will adjust to the new schedule, and it is likely that after several months the entire program will be much less stressful for the patient.

PEDIATRIC RESPIRATORY CARE IN THE HOME

The types of respiratory care prescribed for the pediatric patient in the home are not particularly different from those prescribed for the adult. A child may be prescribed O_2 therapy, aerosol therapy, postural drainage, airway care, mechanical ventilation, and other procedures prescribed for the adult. As with adult home care, pediatric home care can be more cost-effective than hospital care.

Home care for the pediatric patient can involve unique procedures and circumstances. This is most evident in the involvement of the family in providing care for the child and the environment in which the child is developing. Some other differences between pediatric and adult therapy can be the size of equipment, the dosages of medications, such as flow rate of O_2, and the types of equipment used to administer therapy to the child in the home. It is important that home health care for children be flexible and open to input from all those involved. The physician and the health-care providers must be ready to accept alternatives that can improve the effectiveness and efficiency of the therapy provided to the child.

Health-care practitioners performing therapy for a child or training parents should not think of the child as just a "small adult." Gaining cooperation in therapy, satisfying the child's emotional needs, and educating the child require special consideration and patience. Much of the approach to the respiratory care of a pediatric patient depends on the age of the child and the circumstances in the home. There will be little input from a newborn into therapy. But as the child ages, more time will be required for training and education and for input from the child on the effectiveness and monitoring of therapy.

Infant apnea monitoring

One unique aspect of home respiratory care of the child is home apnea monitoring. Each year approximately 7000 children in the United States die from sudden infant death syndrome (SIDS). Most of them die before reaching their first birthday. The majority die between the ages of 3 weeks and 7 months. More children die from SIDS than from cystic fibrosis, childhood cancer, and childhood heart disease put together. It is unclear what causes SIDS. It is not believed to be hereditary, and siblings of SIDS victims do not always exhibit signs of apnea. In many cases a child who appears normal and healthy is found dead in the crib in the morning or after a nap. Autopsies do not reveal the cause of death, but it is not caused by suffocation, aspiration of stomach contents, neglect, or abuse. The children in a wealthy family are equally as likely to die from SIDS as the children in a poor family.

Because the cause of SIDS is unknown, there is no treatment and there are no tests to identify children susceptible to the disorder. Observation of the newborn for symptoms and investigation of family history can help to identify a child who may be "at risk," but there is no set of symptoms that positively identifies a child as a possible SIDS victim. The most common observation is periodic episodes of apnea. Some SIDS victims have been reported to have had a respiratory infection before their death, but this has not been true in all cases. This uncertainty of the cause makes SIDS a puzzling and devastating occurrence in a family. The family's grief and emotional problems after a SIDS death should be considered when treatment, such as monitoring, is instituted for a sibling.

A sleep study can be performed on children suspected of having SIDS to assist in identifying episodes of apnea and to establish a baseline for the child's normal breathing and cardiac pattern. These studies can be conducted in the hospital or at home. If the child demonstrates consistent apnea (periodic episodes of sleep apnea are normal) or the physician suspects that the child may be a SIDS candidate, the child can be monitored at home on an infant apnea monitor. This monitor receives input from an elastic belt or adhesive electrodes placed around the child's upper abdomen and chest. The infant wears these leads at all times of the day and night. The monitor itself is a "box" to which the cable from the leads on the infant is attached. The monitor receives signals from the infant on the child's RR and HR. An alarm sounds if breathing stops for a set period of time or the HR decreases below a set point. Use of an apnea monitor has saved many children from death and their families from the grief of SIDS.

A good home-care company can train parents in the operation of an apnea monitor and should routinely check the function of the equipment. Because most monitors are small and can be battery-powered, the child is not confined to the home. The monitor is worn for as long as the physician believes it is needed, generally until the child is 1 year old.

BIBLIOGRAPHY

Beckett J: Katie Beckett: the little girl who caught the country's eye, AARTimes 9(6):41-43, 56, June 1985.

Bell W et al: Home care and rehabilitation in respiratory medicine, Philadelphia, 1984, JB Lippincott Co.

Connors AF Jr et al: Chest physical therapy: the immediate effect on oxygenation in acutely ill patients, Chest 78(4):559-564, 1980.

Evans GM: SKIP: parents and health care professionals work together for better quality of life, AARTimes 9(6):44-46, June 1985.

Frownfelter DL: Chest physical therapy and pulmonary rehabilitation: an interdisciplinary approach, Chicago, 1978, Year Book Medical Publishers, Inc.

Halmandaris VJ, Cabin W, and McNamara M, editors: Tender loving care: a routine activity with pediatric home care (special issue), Caring 4(5), 1985.

King M: Mucus and mucociliary clearance, Basics RD 11(1):1-7, 1982.

May DB and Munt PW: Physiologic effects of chest percussion and postural drainage in patients with stable chronic bronchitis, Chest 75(1):29-31, 1979.

National Sudden Infant Death Syndrome Foundation: Facts about sudden infant death syndrome, (brochure available from National SIDS Foundation, 2 Metro Plaza, Suite 205, 8240 Professional Place, Landover, MD 20785).

O'Ryan JA and Burns DG: Pulmonary rehabilitation: from hospital to home, 1984, Chicago, Year Book Medical Publishers, Inc.

Pennsylvania Society for Respiratory Therapy, Inc: Respiratory home care procedure manual, Hershey, Pa, 1983, The Society.

Ransom J: Pulmonary home care: your guide to more comfortable breathing, Kansas City, Mo, 1980, Baptist Memorial Hospital.

Rozenberg T: Home care: cleaning of equipment, Respir Ther 67-70, May/June 1973.

Sackner MA: Tracheobronchial toilet, Weekly Update: Pulmonary Medicine 1-8, 1978.

Travenol Laboratories, Inc: Travenol home apnea monitoring program: answers to 12 important questions (brochure), 1985.

Weimer M: Home respiratory therapy for patients with chronic obstructive pulmonary disease, Respir Care 28(11):1484, 1983.

CHAPTER 9

Discharge planning and community resources in pulmonary rehabilitation

THE DISCHARGE PROCESS

A goal of discharge planning is to identify problems the patient may experience and to develop meaningful solutions to those problems. The patient, family, and health-care staff are all essential participants in any discharge plan. Discharge planning should not be done immediately before the patient leaves the hospital. Instead it is a dynamic process carried on throughout the patient's entire hospitalization. The primary objective of the discharge plan is to prepare the patient and family for continuing care after the patient leaves the hospital. To achieve adequate preparation, the discharge plan should take into account both the short- and long-term needs of the patient and family. Following are the four main steps in planning for discharge:

1. Begin the process. Open up channels of communication.
2. Assess the patient and family and their needs and assets.
3. Teach the patient and family about self-care.
4. Plan and implement follow-up.

As part of the medical treatment plan, discharge planning should be initiated as early as possible. It may be that little specific action is required initially, for example, if the patient is in ICU. The time the patient is in ICU can be a valuable opportunity to plan, to educate the family, and to get to know the patient's needs and lifestyle.

Early planning by the health-care team can ensure that communication channels are open between all practitioners and departments involved with the patient, such as respiratory-care services, nursing departments, the hospital's medical social worker, the physician, and the patient and family. Effective communication among the health-care team promotes improved care and initiates the discharge process.

As the director of patient care while the patient is in the acute-care facility and at home, the physician is the major participant in the design of a care program that includes consideration of the patient's needs after discharge. The plan for care and discharge should be based upon established goals and objectives. The specific responsibilities of each team member in the achievement of these goals should be determined. The length of time a patient is expected to spend in the acute-care facility and in need of health care after discharge will influence the goals and objectives established for the patient. It is important that the goals be appropriate to the patient's needs and, moreover, that they be achievable. Goals may need to be revised, and new goals may need to be developed according to the patient's needs.

Patient and family assessment

A thorough care program and discharge plan cannot be developed without an assessment of both the patient and the family. Areas to be evaluated include psychologic (attitude and family relationships), medical (the patient's clinical status and psychomotor abilities), and home environment (physical facilities and the lifestyle of the patient and family). Assessment in each of these areas may require the services of professionals. The team concept in care and discharge planning allows for this input when needed. Determination of a realistic prognosis for the patient promotes better planning and contributes to the establishment of appropriate goals. Through the assessment process, members of the health-care team are able to identify specific areas in which education and training are needed for the patient and family. Education is the first step in preparing the patient and family for the responsibilities of home care, such as administering aerosol therapy, carrying out an exercise program, and performing tracheostomy care.

Preparation of the patient and family for self-care

Providing information to the patient and family about the nature of the patient's illness, the care being provided in the hospital, and any disabilities that may be experienced later is a starting point in preparing for self-care. Eventually, training in specific psychomotor skills and medical care to be administered at home will be addressed. By identifying general and specific objectives in preparation for discharge, the health-care team can make it easier for the patient and family to focus on the information being presented. Some general and specific items that may be included in educational objectives are listed in the box on p. 157.

The overriding goal in preparing for discharge should be developing the confidence of the patient and family in their own competence to provide self-care. Promoting this confidence should always be in the minds of health-care personnel. It is important to take advantage of opportunities to reinforce confidence through encouragement, explanation of procedures, and skills practice.

Follow-up after discharge

A thorough, consistent follow-up program after discharge assures the patient and family that they have not been abandoned. It can contribute to improved compliance with a home-care program. Too often, follow-up involves only the physician or the physician's office staff. The relationships that have been developed during the patient's stay in the acute-care facility are valuable and should be continued after the patient is discharged.

It is not possible to prepare a patient for every situation that may occur after

_____ **EDUCATIONAL OBJECTIVES FOR DISCHARGE** _____

General

Understanding of the rationale for therapy
Ability to control symptoms and to recognize warning signs of problems
Understanding of the patient's limitations and abilities
Understanding of the disease and the resulting disabilities

Specific

Detailed description of procedures to be performed
Operation, maintenance, and care of equipment
Demonstration of competence in therapy administration
Personalization of information to the home setting from general instruction
Written instructions for all procedures

discharge, but open, continuous communication with the patient allows professional input regarding problems as they occur. Staff members in the hospital or rehabilitation program are often more accessible than the physician. The staff can often contact the physician if a problem requires immediate attention more quickly than the patient can. At times the patient may not consider a change in a symptom significant enough to mention to the physician. The patient may feel more comfortable asking the professional opinion of another member of the health-care team. The patient can be urged to contact the physician about the change in symptoms when the patient may not have otherwise. In addition, the patient's observation and self-assessment skills can be confirmed and strengthened, and a notation can be made on the patient's rehabilitation and home-care record.

Follow-up after acute care allows the patient to personalize further the material presented in the hospital. The information and skills acquired in the acute-care facility can be reinforced, and new material or skills can be presented as necessary. Follow-up that is initiated by the health-care team makes a statement about the relationship that has been established with the patient. A phone call or a letter lets the patient know there is access to professional help. Because the physician's office is the most frequent location for follow-up, it is important that the office staff be familiar with the care plan, discharge plan, and course of events during the patient's hospitalization.

MEDICAL PERSONNEL AND THEIR ROLES IN PLANNING FOR DISCHARGE

Discharge planning, like other aspects of health care, is a team effort. The best planning for discharge takes place when the skills and knowledge of every professional available to the patient are included. The box on p. 158 lists some health professionals and the tasks they would perform in discharge planning.

POSSIBLE ROLES OF THE HEALTH-CARE TEAM IN DISCHARGE

Physician

Supervision of all aspects of the final discharge plan

Prescription of care in the hospital and at home

Communication with other members of the health-care team about the patient's condition and discharge status

Input into content of educational material

Education on and reinforcement of self-care

Education of the members of the discharge team

Respiratory-care personnel

Instruction on respiratory-therapy equipment and treatments

Tracheostomy care, suctioning, instruction in anatomy and physiology, and pathophysiology of disease

Explanation of rationale for treatments, monitoring of response, maximizing of self-administration of therapy

Nursing personnel

ICU and floor nurses: reinforcing proper self-care techniques and other aspects of general respiratory care, such as hygiene, assessment of symptoms, special medical needs, etc.

Education about medications: names, actions, side effects, and dosages

Medical social worker

Communication with the patient about insurance requirements, financial needs, social agencies, and community resources

Psychologic assessment and identification of needs and resources to meet them

Arranging for home-care needs, equipment, personnel, and modifications to deal with disabilities

Other health-care personnel

Occupational therapist, physical therapist, nurse-specialist, rehabilitation staff, nutritionist, and psychiatrist or counselor

Perform duties according to the needs and medical problems of the patient.

Patient and family education in discharge planning

Education and training of the patient and family make up the cornerstone of a positive discharge experience. Education provides the foundation for the development of self-confidence in the patient. It allows for identification of the patient's needs and individualization of any program designed to meet these needs. The support of the family or other people involved with the patient is crucial to successful recovery and self-care. In many instances poor response to out-patient treatment is the result of a lack of a support network in the patient's life. Educating all persons concerned about the patient promotes consistency and coordination in the comprehensive care of the pulmonary patient. Identification of a tentative discharge date allows for good planning and organization of the material to be presented. This planning and organization requires effective communication among the health professionals on the team.

COMMUNITY RESOURCES

Numerous resources exist in the community to help the patient cope with disabilities and other problems. Many of these resources are available to promote independent function, to maximize functional ability, to train the patient to achieve a specific objective, or to provide needed equipment. Following are some possible problem areas for the patient and family. Assistance in many of these areas can be attained by identifying and using the appropriate community resource.

Financial

Emotional and psychologic

Family and marital

Nutritional

Social isolation

Educational and informational

Follow-up care in the home

Occupational

Equipment needs

The hospital social worker or discharge planner is usually responsible for identifying patient needs and for coordinating access to community resources. If the social worker or discharge planner can become involved with the patient well before discharge, interaction with the patient and family will be improved. This improved interaction promotes a more thorough and professional understanding of the patient's needs and the appropriate resources to meet them.

Where to get information on social-service agencies

In settings in which there is no discharge planner or medical social worker, it may be difficult to find out what resources are available and how to gain access to them. In such cases health-care providers can over time develop a list of the major resources found in the community and distribute it to the patient and family. The patient and family can then investigate for themselves the resources they believe will be beneficial to them after discharge. The box on p. 160 lists some of the most common community resources. The best possible situation for all concerned exists when a match can be made between the needs of the patient and the resources available. It should be remembered that social-service agencies exist to help people meet their needs and that these agencies want people to take advantage of their services.

--- **SOURCES OF INFORMATION ON COMMUNITY RESOURCES** ---

The "Help Book" in many communities lists social services, volunteer agencies, and other programs in the community.

County welfare offices, health services, and services for the elderly

Social Security Administration (Numerous pamphlets are available to explain services and assist in filing claims.)

Profit-making agencies (listed in the Yellow Pages under social-service organizations)

United Way

Physician or other member of the health-care team

Local chapters of medical societies and professional organizations

State Department of Vocational Rehabilitation and employment services, such as the Labor Department

Community mental-health centers

Local churches

Transportation and meals may be available through Meals on Wheels or Senior Wheels.

The Medic Alert Foundation provides engraved necklaces, wristbands, etc. to alert others to the patient's needs.

A list of paramedic and ambulance services should be compiled.

State and local chapters (Christmas Seal offices) of the American Lung Association

Visiting-nurse agencies

Nonprofit organizations associated with a specific disease, such as cystic fibrosis, asthma, or cancer

Occasionally the patient is reluctant to accept "help" from an available source because of cultural or personal reasons. Some people are uncomfortable using public or private money for their own needs. Others prefer to be self-reliant and therefore find accepting help difficult. The decision to accept help belongs to the patient and the patient's right to refuse it should be respected. Following are some strategies for encouraging the patient and family to accept help:

1. Provide several alternatives for each situation. (There usually is more than one solution to a problem.)
2. Allow the patient to think over the whole situation and talk to a friend or family member before deciding.
3. Have the patient meet someone who has used the services. Many home-care companies can suggest someone.
4. Solicit support from the physician for the patient's involvement with the community resource.
5. Provide a trial period. Let the patient explore various alternatives. Let the patient know that a decision does not constitute a long-term commitment and that if the situation changes in the future or the patient is not satisfied, the patient may consider other options.

How to seek help

Frequently the patient and family will have difficulty with the search for help, especially if they have never used community services in the past. Organizing the effort to seek services that meet the patient's needs helps the family get started. Several steps have been found to be helpful in organizing and keeping the search focused.

The patient or family member exploring community resources should *have the specific problem (need) stated in writing.* It should be written clearly in nonmedical terms. The patient or family member should ask, "What is the help I am seeking?" A discharge planner or member of the health-care team can help define the need. By defining the need, the patient or family member keeps from getting sidetracked to other "good ideas" and helps the agency providing assistance to understand the need and to direct the seeker to the appropriate people.

It is important that the patient and family realize that finding out exactly what resources are available will require a considerable amount of time. A great deal of the frustration that often occurs during this process can be prevented if the patient or family member is prepared to spend the necessary time. Having information in writing helps to keep the frustration level as low as possible. *The search for assistance in the community is a learning process.* The patient and family will get better at it with practice.

Networking among the agencies in the community is a good way to organize the search for information about services. If an organization that is contacted for help is not able to meet the need, the patient should ask that agency for another source of help. When another agency or person is recommended, ask the referring agency what questions should be asked to get to the point and to help the recommended agency understand the need. Ask the referring individual if the explanation was clear and if enough information was given. The patient or family member should always *make notes of the conversation, whether it was conducted over the phone or in person.* The patient or family member should write down the name of each person spoken to, the phone numbers called, and the essential comments or information obtained. The patient or family member should ask for qualitative as well as quantitative information and find out if the agency can give the name and phone number of anyone else who has used the service. The patient or family member should ask for handouts or other written material from the agency about its services and should ask to be put on the agency's mailing list if it has one. Before visiting an agency or office, the patient or family member should find out specifically what information will be required during the visit. *All records, numbers, names, dates, and forms should be readily accessible.*

The best attitude to have during the search for help is that of a learner. A good deal of patience is needed. The patient or family member should ask for an explanation of any unfamiliar terms or concepts to increase knowledge and understanding of the system. If there is uncertainty about what was said, the patient or family member should ask that it be repeated, write it down, then repeat it back to make sure it is correct. If the person to whom the patient or family member is speaking is not able to answer questions satisfactorily, the patient or family member should call again on another day or ask to speak to someone else about the problem. After receiving the desired help or the answers to questions, it is a good practice to write a letter to the individual who helped. The patient or family member should pleasantly and positively let the agency know that it has been helpful.

PSYCHOSOCIAL ASPECTS OF DISCHARGE

Whether in the acute-care facility or at home, the patient has psychologic and emotional needs. This aspect of patient care is not consciously ignored in any given health-care situation, but the urgency of acute physical problems may decrease the opportunity for the staff to meet psychosocial and emotional needs. The psychosocial aspect of care is influenced by all health-care practitioners coming into contact with the patient or the patient's family. The attitudes of the members of the health-care team toward the patient, the prognosis, and the effectiveness of the care plan are communicated to the patient and family. These attitudes affect greatly the atmosphere of any health-care situation, whether in-patient or out-patient. They can also influence the quality of self-care performed at home.

Being aware of some of the psychologic and emotional problems a patient may experience can help health-care providers to recognize problems when they arise and to assist the patient whenever possible. Some of the psychosocial and emotional concerns expressed by many patients with a chronic disability, such as COPD, are listed below:

Anxiety and fear of suffocation
Loss of control over the patient's life
Unwanted role and lifestyle changes
Depression, withdrawal, and isolation
Few social and physical outlets
Loss of self-esteem

Common problems experienced by patients with COPD

Fear of suffocation is a major problem for the patient with a pulmonary disorder. The sensation of dyspnea is a signal to the patient of the surpassing of physical limits. Panic and the feeling of being out of control are common when dyspnea is severe. The patient must gain confidence in his ability to recognize his limits, especially his tolerance to physical exertion. Using the techniques involved in desensitization to dyspnea can be very helpful in gaining this confidence (see ventilation retraining, Chapter 4).

Loss of control over the patient's own life and destiny is also a major concern for many patients. In some ways the traditional health-care system contributes to this feeling of loss of control by encouraging dependence and passive behavior in the patient in the acute-care facility. The patient often feels like the disease is in control,

SAMPLE QUESTIONS FROM THE BECK DEPRESSION INVENTORY
(SHORT FORM)* (2 OF 13 QUESTIONS ON THE SCALE)

D. (Dissatisfaction)

3 I am dissatisfied with everything.
2 I don't get satisfaction out of anything anymore.
1 I don't enjoy things the way I used to.
0 I am not particularly dissatisfied.

I. (Indecisiveness)

3 I can't make any decisions at all anymore.
2 I have great difficulty in making decisions.
1 I try to put off making decisions.
0 I make decisions about as well as ever.

*Items from the Beck Depression Inventory. Copyright © 1987 by Beck AT, MD. Reproduced by permission of publisher, The Psychological Corporation. All rights reserved.

setting limits to behavior and causing changes in relationships and roles in life. A sense of control and responsibility can be developed over time as the patient reestablishes a lifestyle that recognizes the patient's disabilities and strives to maximize the patient's potential within objective limits.

Changes in traditional roles and lifestyle can be significant to the patient with a pulmonary disorder. New skills may have to be developed to enable the patient to adjust to new roles and lifestyle patterns. Few people are prepared for the major adjustments required by a chronic illness. The patient needs to develop an understanding of the disease and the relationship between the disease and the disabilities it causes. Acceptance of the new circumstances promotes development of skills for dealing with various aspects of the disabilities. Finally, the patient needs to acknowledge the need for help in certain circumstances and to know how to obtain this help.

Depression, perhaps the most common experience of patients with a chronic disability, can be difficult to identify and address in the plan for care or discharge. Health-care practitioners can have a positive influence on the patient in this area by demonstrating a willingness to listen and a genuine interest in the patient. At times it is difficult for a patient to talk about problems and feelings. The short form of the Beck Depression Inventory (see box above) can be a useful instrument in assessing the existence of depression and the level of depression a patient may be experiencing. Two examples of the statements on the Beck Depression Inventory are given in the box above.

This instrument can be administered quickly and easily in the physician's office or at the rehabilitation facility. It allows the health-care staff to "quantify" the patient's feelings and may warn the staff of the existence of severe depression. Severe depression is often not as obvious to the untrained observer as one might believe. Its presence certainly affects patient compliance and participation in rehabilitation and self-care activities.

When the patient first examines his situation (having a chronic disability), it may seem that there are few social outlets. Society is improving its recognition of the humanness of the disabled, but there is room for further improvement. Theaters, stadiums, museums, schools, restaurants, and other public places are being made more accessible to the handicapped. Alternative activities for the patient and the patient's attitude toward attending regular activities and functions should be discussed. An inquiry into why the patient believes he should or should not be involved in social activities will open a discussion of the patient's fears and concerns. It is also an opportunity to identify areas of interest. (Appendix D can also be helpful in identifying these areas.) The patient can learn that social isolation is not a necessary outcome of a chronic disability.

The loss of self-esteem that accompanies a major disability can affect all other aspects of a care program. The patient must feel worthy, or expending the tremendous effort required in rehabilitation activities will be difficult. The patient should be encouraged to look away from himself to the people around him for opportunities to help. Health-care practitioners can help by pointing out genuine contributions that can be made by the patient. The patient may not see his new contributions as significant, especially if they are different from previous behavior. Services such as house-sitting, baby-sitting, cleaning, making phone calls, and planning are only a few possibilities. The patient should be encouraged to develop hobbies and to look for opportunities to participate in family and public life.

A positive attitude from the health-care practitioners involved with the patient is important, but at times such an attitude is difficult to maintain and can be emotionally draining for the staff. Staff meetings should include opportunities to discuss the attitudes surrounding patient care and should provide an outlet for frustration and other staff concerns. *A genuinely positive attitude and a willingness to listen are often the best short-term help that can be offered to the patient in need.*

The family and other people who are significant to the patient also have a major effect on the psychosocial wellness of the patient. Involving the family in program activities and routine discussions can help the patient and family cope with the disabilities and lifestyle changes caused by the disorder. The family must be made to feel that they are part of the health-care team. If they do feel this way, they will develop a realistic understanding of the disabilities and limitations involved in the disorder and gain an appreciation of the contribution they can make to patient care.

Development and resolution of a crisis

When does a physical, psychosocial, or emotional problem for a patient become a medical one requiring immediate medical intervention? Both in the hospital and at home, the answer to this question often depends on whether or not the patient feels there is a crisis. Has the level of stress, physical and emotional, reached a point beyond which the patient believes can be managed? For some people this excessive stress may be experienced only during emergencies, but for other people the excessive stress has built up over time or develops from many different sources coming together. In either case the crisis is a tremendous threat to the patient.

Hearing a diagnosis of emphysema, chronic bronchitis, cancer, or other disease is psychologically and emotionally devastating to many people. Adjustment to this situation is not an easy or simple process. Admission to a hospital or even seeking medical help in a physician's office is not routine. Often the reason help is being sought is that the individual is in a crisis, a situation that is out of control, and is unable to deal with it independently. Crisis is an alarming word, and its meaning here could include the extremes of physical, psychologic, or emotional problems. More often the crisis referred to here may be transient or relatively mild in degree (low in intensity but long in duration). The development of an emotional crisis and at times the precipitation of a physical crisis can be influenced by the following four aspects of the patient's life:

Perception of the problem

Resources available

Specific stressor involved

Previous behaviors developed for coping with stress

The more the patient perceives the physical change or symptom experienced as a major problem, the greater the likelihood that a crisis will develop. What one patient perceives as a major change in typical symptoms, another patient may view as a minor inconvenience. A change in sputum color may be of little concern to a patient, especially if the patient is used to this occurring. But the patient may become alarmed if blood is found in the sputum and SOB and fatigue are felt more quickly than usual.

If good resources are available to enable the patient to deal with the problem independently, the problem is less likely to grow into a crisis situation. Some possible resources are family members or other significant people in the patient's life who are available and can reassure the patient. The availability of financial resources and the accessibility of a physician, other health-care practitioner, or an acute-care facility can all influence the development of a crisis.

The specific symptom or aspect of the patient's life that is producing the stress (the stressor) has a major influence on the development and severity of a crisis. Persistent, severe chest pain radiating to the left arm and jaw is likely to be thought of as more significant than transient SOB experienced after walking up a flight of stairs. The loss of a loved one, especially one who assisted the patient in self-care, may cause a crisis for the patient.

Throughout life each person develops methods of coping with all the various difficulties that arise. Some persons develop more and deeper coping mechanisms than others, especially if they had not been sheltered from trials and tribulations. A patient who has experienced a symptom in the past usually has developed some means of dealing with the problem. In general the less experience an individual has in dealing with a problem and being responsible for the solution, the more poorly the person will handle a stressful situation.

If situations that have the potential to develop into crises for the patient can be identified, appropriate means of intervention can be taught. This intervention may involve modifying the stressor, altering the perception of the problem, or developing coping mechanisms. It is important to begin the process of resolving a developing or existing crisis as early as possible to minimize the effect of the problem on the long-term situation.

The physical disabilities and discomfort caused by a disorder are closely linked to the patient's psychologic and emotional state. It is important that the physical problems being experienced be dealt with effectively, especially if they are severe or acute. Prompt attention to physical problems helps the patient and the health-care team to focus on the effect of the problems on the psychologic or emotional aspects of patient care.

Resolution of a psychologic or emotional crisis occurs over time and in recognizable steps. Initially the patient experiencing the crisis, such as a recent diagnosis of emphysema or the first admission to the emergency room (ER) with SOB, may feel shocked, anxious, or helpless by the realization of what is happening. This realization can be extremely frightening for the patient, and the patient may at times border on panic. After a time the patient may become defensive. The defensiveness often appears as anger, at the patient himself or at others, or a frank denial of the symptoms being experienced. At some point during the resolution of the problems, the patient will accept the reality of the symptoms and the disorder. Once the patient is able to acknowledge it, the problem can be discussed and dealt with constructively. As the patient begins to adapt to the new situation, the disorder, and the subsequent disabilities, constructive ways of coping can be sought. The patient is most educable at this point and may be open to suggestions for rehabilitation and changes in behavior. If a health-care practitioner can determine the point a patient is at in resolving the problem, the practitioner can be supportive, making communication more effective. As part of the multidisciplinary health-care team, professional mental-health counselors should be contacted when appropriate. Counselors may be involved directly in discussions with the patient, or they may train the staff to talk with the patient and family. This training may also include recognizing problems and improvements in mental status. The health-care practitioner in contact with the patient can be a valuable asset in helping the patient to move toward the more open, adaptive stages of crisis resolution.

METHODS OF INTERVENTION BY HEALTH-CARE PRACTITIONERS

What can the typical health-care practitioner do to help a patient with psychosocial and emotional problems? When the patient and family are seen for such a short period of time during a hospitalization, can the health-care practitioner make any contribution?

Observe the patient and family for both verbal and nonverbal behavior that may indicate the need for help and the type of help needed. Look for appropriate opportunities for intervention by professional counselors, such as when the family is visiting, and alert the counseling staff. It is also helpful if the health-care practitioner asks herself several questions: Is the patient oriented to time and space? How do the patient and family answer questions and give information? How does the patient verbally express feelings to the staff and other people in the room? Does the patient express interest in activity outside the room and in the world in general?

Listen to the patient and family when they speak to you and to each other. Give the patient an opportunity to express himself verbally in a nonthreatening, sincere, and relaxed manner. Ask open-ended questions of the patient and family. Bring up the subject of feelings and thoughts about their situation and the care they are receiving. They may not want to talk at a certain time, but groundwork for later discussions can be laid. Make yourself vulnerable, especially to rejection by the patient. Showing vulnerability is important because it can communicate your own human nature and your empathy for the patient and family's situation. If a patient or family member does not wish to talk to a particular health-care worker, find out whom the person would be willing to talk to and arrange for the two people to get together. If the patient wishes to talk about a certain topic, arrange an opportunity to discuss it, no matter what the topic may be. No subject should be considered inappropriate. If you are not comfortable or competent in dealing with an issue, make an effort to find someone who will be able to help the patient.

Give positive reinforcement whenever possible. Recognize the patient's small improvements and efforts. Do not let an opportunity for encouragement go by simply because you think it is too small to be important. Comment on objective improvements in the performance of ADL, especially when independence is demonstrated. But do not make things up or build them up to be greater than they are; sincerity is very important. A COPD patient is likely to feel "down" because little objective physical improvement can be seen. From the patient's perspective the future holds only further deterioration and disability. By pointing out small steps toward increased function in ADL, this attitude can be improved.

Education plays an important role in helping the patient adjust to his situation. Information about his condition can alleviate many fears and misunderstandings and foster in the patient a greater sense of control and independence. Whether or not it is verbalized, it is likely that the patient has thought about the future and what the new realities will mean. Some of the issues that can be discussed are nervousness in social situations, ways to relax, development of a positive self-concept, fear of suffocation, breathing retraining, and use of medications.

Documentation of all significant conversations and comments is a valuable aid to the physician and to any counseling professional who becomes involved with the patient and family. A record of comments should include any changes, positive or negative. This record can be helpful during follow-up and assessment of progress toward social and emotional adjustment. Health-care practitioners should seek clarification of "off-the-cuff" comments from the patient or family. These findings should become part of the patient's record, especially as an aid to formal professional counseling.

Referral to professional counseling is important, especially for problems identified by the staff that cannot be handled through the normal mechanisms of a health-care program. Poor compliance, persistent depression, and lack of verbal communication may indicate a need for professional help. Whenever serious problems are identified or problems seem to linger, professional counseling should be sought.

Counseling can help the patient and family to put their concerns and feelings into words. It can contribute to a realistic appraisal of the patient's condition, functional capacity, and prospects for change. Many mental-health workers may not be familiar with all the physical details of a particular disorder. It is important that the health-care staff involved with the patient communicate with the counselor during the counseling process. A list of social-service and mental-health counseling services should be maintained as a referral list for use by the health-care staff. Over time, communication about and understanding of psychosocial problems will benefit the entire health-care team.

BIBLIOGRAPHY

American Hospital Association: Common social and emotional problems, Staff manual for teaching patients about COPD, Chapter 2: Psychosocial issues, 71-76, 1982, The Association.

Beck AT and Beck RW: Screening depressed patients in family practice: a rapid technic, Postgrad Med 52:81-85, Dec 1972.

Cronin MP: Home care: taking full advantage of voluntary associations, Respir Ther 35, March/April 1977.

Dudley DL et al: Psychosocial concomitants to rehabilitation in chronic obstructive pulmonary disease, Part 1: Psychosocial and psychological considerations, Chest 77(3):413-420, 1980.

Dudley DL et al: Psychosocial concomitants to rehabilitation in chronic obstructive pulmonary disease, Part 2: Psychosocial treatment, Chest 77(4):544-551, 1980.

Dudley DL et al: Psychosocial concomitants to rehabilitation in chronic obstructive pulmonary disease, Part 3: Dealing with psychiatric disease (as distinguished from psychosocial or psychophysiologic problems), Chest 77(5):677-684, 1980.

Hodgkin JE, Zorn E, and Connors G: Pulmonary rehabilitation: guidelines to success, Stoneham, Mass, 1984, Butterworth Publishers.

O'Ryan JA and Burns DG: Pulmonary rehabilitation: from hospital to home, Chicago, 1984, Year Book Medical Publishers, Inc.

Petty TL et al: Community resources for rehabilitation of patients with chronic obstructive pulmonary diseases and cor pulmonale (pulmonary rehabilitation study group), Circulation Volume XLIX A1-A20, Washington, DC, May 1974, US Government Printing Office.

Zung WW: A self-rating depression scale, Arch Gen Psychiatry 12:63-70, Jan 1965.

CHAPTER 10

The home-care company and durable medical equipment in home care

CONTINUITY OF CARE

For the patient with a pulmonary disorder, a program of home respiratory care is an extension of the visit to the physician's office, hospitalization, or involvement in a pulmonary rehabilitation program. Home care may be a continuation of the treatments and therapies received in the hospital, but it can also involve new treatments, exercises, and therapies. It is difficult to reinforce new respiratory-care techniques outside a formal setting. A home-care company can be a valuable ally in reinforcement of therapy, assessment, and patient follow-up, but the home-care company and the equipment supplier are often overlooked as community resources.

Compliance with a self-care program after discharge from the hospital or rehabilitation program or after leaving the physician's office can be enhanced in several ways. One way is to establish an individualized program of activities with specific, measurable goals so the patient knows exactly what to do and what results to expect. A second method is to arrange for frequent follow-up, including a review of goals and revision of program activities as the patient's condition changes. When activities are revised, the home-care program is dynamic, and the health-care process is continuing. Not every patient will require an extensive home-care program. By establishing a well thought-out, clearly understood guide for the patient, the financial and the psychologic and physical aspects of care can be controlled. A home-care company can play an important role in home respiratory care.

THE ROLE OF A DURABLE MEDICAL EQUIPMENT (DME) COMPANY IN HOME RESPIRATORY CARE

A weak link in the health care of many patients is follow-up to prescribed therapy. Without follow-up, patient compliance suffers, and ultimately the patient and the health-care system also suffer. For the patient requiring O_2 equipment or other ancillary medical equipment for home use, the DME company can be of assistance. Occasionally a visiting nurse is required to perform some skilled nursing care for the homebound patient with a pulmonary disorder, but skilled nursing care more often is not necessary. When a patient is using O_2 in the home, the regular visits from the representative of the home-care company provide an opportunity for follow-up.

There has been a significant increase in the number of medical-equipment suppliers and home-care companies in recent years. Home-care companies often have grown out of existing DME companies that recognized the need for delivery of health-care services in the home. Numerous respiratory-care practitioners have seen home care as a new opportunity for professional growth. Their movement into this area of care has created a pool of trained personnel to provide high-quality care and service in the home. The DME company often provides patient-care services and education along with the medical equipment.

A good home-care company can be a tremendous asset to a health-care team. Many forms of pulmonary care can be performed safely and effectively in the home by the individual or family, and home care usually is less expensive than hospital care. A number of home-care companies have established home ventilator services and assessment programs for reporting the status of the patient to the physician. The routine visits to the patient's home to assess the operation of equipment can be an opportunity to reinforce the care plan in the home environment. Regular communication with the patient's physician and other members of the rehabilitation team improves the flow of information about the effectiveness of the program. It also provides for a check on the patient's compliance with the prescribed self-care program.

The patient contributes to her own health care by performing the prescribed care techniques and by making suggestions about the care program. The patient can teach the members of the health-care team about alternative ways of giving care in the home and about which care techniques work best for the patient. Communication among the health-care team begins with education of the patient and family and can be enhanced greatly by a home-care company. The company can act as a conduit between the patient and the health-care team for information and data that may not otherwise have been transmitted.

At times it is difficult for the patient to understand fully the medications and instructions given upon discharge. The patient often has questions once at home and beginning to carry out the physician's orders. Many patients may be reluctant to call the physician if they have a "small" question or if they are unclear about when or how often a therapy, medication, or exercise should be administered or performed. For these and other reasons, the patient does not properly comply with the prescribed care plan. Having a qualified health-care practitioner visit the patient in the home environment to provide further instruction, encouragement, and assessment of the patient's situation can have a tremendous effect on the effectiveness of the medical care provided by the physician.

Quality in a home-care provider

Health-care practitioners are often asked to recommend a home-care or DME company. With the recent growth in the number of such companies, it is difficult to be familiar with the strengths and weaknesses of each one. DME companies have not historically been expected to provide patient-care services. But because of current competition and need, the provision of health-care services by DME companies and the need for knowledgeable providers is increasing. The box on p. 172 lists some suggested criteria against which to measure a home-care company. A company possessing these characteristics would be able to participate as a valued member of the health-care team.

These criteria place a great deal of emphasis on patient-care skills rather than simply equipment supply and assembly. The companies need to provide follow-up, education, and quality respiratory care to maintain the status as contributing members of the health-care team. It is a challenge for many home-care providers to strive for the highest possible level of professionalism in respiratory care at home. The Joint Commission on Accreditation of Health Care Organizations (JCAHCO) has established accreditation standards for home-care companies. They now offer accreditation to home-care providers just as hospitals are accredited.

GUIDELINES FOR PROVIDERS OF O_2 SYSTEMS

It is the responsibility of the home-care company to ensure that all respiratory-therapy equipment placed in the home is working properly before being installed. The box on p. 173 contains a list of suggested equipment that may be installed by a home-care company in the home of a patient for whom an O_2 concentrator has been prescribed.

The home-care company must also see that all federal and state regulations concerning use of O_2 and medical equipment are being adhered to by its staff and the patient. Vehicles transporting O_2 cylinders must be properly labeled according to Department of Transportation (DOT) standards. All National Fire Protection Association (NFPA) and Compressed Gas Association (CGA) guidelines should be strictly adhered to during storage and handling of O_2 in cylinders and liquid reservoirs.

Before equipment is delivered to a patient's home, an attempt to arrange for a delivery time, such as between 2 and 4 PM, should be made. By establishing a range of time for delivery, all interested parties can be present, and personnel scheduling is simplified. It is best if the delivery time allows the patient and/or the persons who will be responsible for the equipment to be present. During equipment installation, it should be explained that a follow-up visit to the home will be made, usually within 24 to 48 hours of the patient's arrival at home, and that it will provide an opportunity to review equipment operation.

SUGGESTED CRITERIA FOR PROVIDERS OF RESPIRATORY HOME CARE

1. A qualified, credentialed respiratory-care practitioner on-call 24 hours per day
2. Qualified, credentialed full-time employees providing respiratory care (trained in patient assessment, pulmonary-rehabilitation modalities, and equipment usage)
3. A minimum of one visit (about 1 hour in length) per month (more frequent visits when indicated, documentation sent to the physician)
4. Verbal and written instructions provided at the time any equipment is set up in the home (written procedures, jargon-free, provided for the operation and cleaning of all equipment, including hazards, precautions, and safety information)
5. Follow-up visit and/or instruction provided 48 to 72 hours after the initial setup of equipment in the home
6. A written record of quality control and maintenance for all equipment
7. A full line of equipment provided and an adequate supply of different O_2 systems, respiratory-care equipment and disposable items (such as cylinders, liquid, concentrators, and suction) maintained
8. Large-capacity "backup" O_2 system provided to patients using a concentrator
9. Transportable O_2 systems available for patients using a concentrator
10. Written report of interview questions, patient-assessment criteria, and equipment-checking procedures done for each visit
11. Full disclosure and review of all charges to the patient before equipment is set up
12. Social worker/counselor knowledgeable in community resources and paperwork available in company office
13. Written policy and procedures for collection of the portion of charges not covered completely by third-party payers
14. Written policy and procedures (such as decision criteria and chain of authority) for handling emergency situations
15. Designated medical advisor/director (nonowner) to the company
16. Written policy and procedures for all equipment and patient use of equipment
17. Written and verbal follow-up provided to the referral source
18. Coordination of services with other health-care providers (when patient receives care from more than one source)
19. Responsibility for notifying the local fire department and electrical company of O_2 or life-support equipment requiring electricity being used in the home
20. Maintenance of a familiarity with up-to-date supplies and equipment available to meet all patient needs
21. Program of in-service/continuing education to keep staff updated on new equipment and procedures

---

A visit to the patient's home by a representative of the home-care company should be arranged within 48 hours of the patient's arrival at home to reinforce the material presented during equipment installation. Copies of the patient assessment and the check-off sheet for installation should be sent to the physician ordering the therapy. These documents can be placed in the patient's medical record to assure the physician that orders are being followed.

It is important that the company installing the equipment place a call to the power

_____ **EXAMPLES OF O₂ THERAPY EQUIPMENT PLACED IN THE HOME** _____

1 O₂ concentrator
1 Gas humidifier, bubbler
2 6-foot lengths of O₂ connecting tubing*‡
1 Connector for O₂ connecting tubing*‡
1 Cannula, such as Laurette style-Flare tip†
1 Backup K or M cylinder
1 Regulator for K or M cylinder
1 Floor stand for large cylinder
1 Aluminum E cylinder for ambulation
1 Cart for E cylinder
1 Regulator for E cylinder

*Extra lengths of tubing and connectors may be required to allow the patient to perform ADL in the home.
†Three additional cannulas should be given for weekly changes. The patient should dispose of the old cannulas.
‡Additional connecting tubing and connectors should be given to the patient to equal the initial setup length. This additional tubing should be used to replace soiled connecting tubing when needed or at least every 2 weeks. The entire length of connecting tubing should be changed by the patient, and the importance of secure connections between the tubing sections should be emphasized.

company supplying electricity to the patient's home and to the fire station closest to the patient's home to notify them of the presence of O₂-therapy equipment in the home and the need for priority treatment in the event of an emergency. Whenever possible, training of the patient and family should begin while the patient is in the acute-care facility. This training can be done by the staff of the acute-care facility or by the staff of the home-care company.

DME COMPANY PROCEDURES FOR INSTALLATION OF O₂ EQUIPMENT

Presentation of a professional image by the home-care provider is important to instill confidence and establish a professional relationship among the patient, the family, and the company. It is possible that a patient requiring O₂ therapy for a long period of time may see the staff of the home-care company, who may be visiting on a monthly basis, more often than the patient sees the physician.

Upon arrival at the patient's home, it is courteous to park the company vehicle in the street and not in the patient's driveway. Before entering the home, introduce yourself, make sure your name tag is visible, and mention the ordering physician's name and the company's name. The patient and family may wish to make a phone call to confirm your identity. This practice should not be discouraged. Explain your purpose for being there, and request permission to inspect the home before placement

ITEMS TO BE NOTED IN THE PATIENT'S HOME
BEFORE INSTALLING EQUIPMENT

1. Location and number of electrical outlets, electrical appliances in the room and the circuit in the home on which the equipment may be operating
2. The number and location of heating ducts, registers, or heating elements in the area where equipment will be placed
3. Entrances and exits to the room and home, such as windows and doors, and the location of large pieces of furniture
4. An interview with the patient or others about ADL. Keep in mind the patient's mobility during recovery.
5. Distance to bedside commode, bathroom, closets, chairs, television, and dressers in the room
6. Rearrange the furniture as little as possible, but select an accessible, appropriate location for the concentrator and/or cylinders.

Remember

Keep cylinders and the tubing carrying the gas at least 10 feet away from direct sunlight, sources of heat, sparks, or open flames.

Avoid placing equipment in entrances and exits to the area and in other high-traffic locations.

Consider all possibilities for "snagging" the O_2 connecting tubing. Keep it out of the way.

Do not store cylinders or other O_2 equipment in a confined space, such as a closet.

The back-up cylinder does not need to be adjacent to the concentrator or the patient, but it certainly should be within the same area.

---

of the equipment. (Guidelines for inspection are listed in the box above.) Try to rearrange the furniture in the home as little as possible. Giving literature on the equipment to the patient and family as the equipment is being set up provides an opportunity for them to read and ask questions.

When delivering equipment into the home, use every opportunity to teach the patient and family about the equipment and its operation. Place the concentrator and cylinder in the agreed-upon location. Attach the humidifier, O_2 connecting tube, and cannula to the concentrator. Plug in the concentrator, but do not turn it on yet. The time when equipment is being set up and checked out is an excellent opportunity for patient and family instruction. If the patient is present, the O_2 from the device will be needed. Keep in mind that the equipment will need to be turned off at some point to allow for a thorough explanation and practice. This will require some planning, but it can certainly be accomplished by using the system being installed. Make sure that the cylinder stand is around the cylinder and that it is secure. Warn the patient and family of the noise, then crack the cylinder valve, connect the regulator securely to the cylinder, and check its operation. Close the cylinder and drain all pressure from the regulator. Replace any furniture that was disturbed when the equipment was placed in the room. Post "No smoking" signs at the entrance to the area and near the equipment. Clean up any loose waste material from the area and request that the patient and family assemble for instruction.

The box on p. 176 gives some of the safety procedures to be followed by the home-care company when storing and handling O_2 cylinders.

Instructing the patient and family

Chapter 3 reviews in detail the principles to be followed and the topics to be covered in a program of education for the patient and family. The emphasis of the instruction at this time is the O_2 equipment to be used by the patient in the home (see boxes on pp. 49 and 178).

It is possible that the patient has never been told about the O_2 prescription, but it is imperative that the physician's order be explained in detail. This should include the O_2 flow rate (in liters per minute) to be used, the times it is to be used, and any specific instructions from the physician, such as to use O_2 only with activity. If the O_2 is to be used intermittently, explain the exact number of hours per day it is to be used. Be sure to demonstrate and explain how to read the flowmeter and the gauge indicating cylinder content. Emphasize to all persons concerned with the patient that no other flow rate should be used without consulting the physician.

A brief review or explanation of what O_2 is and what it is not may be in order. Explain that O_2 is *not* flammable or explosive but that it supports burning; therefore flammable items, such as clothing, burn more quickly in the presence of O_2. For this reason, no smoking or open flames should be permitted when O_2 is in use. A general guideline from the NFPA is that a flame or heat source should be no closer to an O_2 source than 10 feet. This includes the tubing through which the gas travels and the concentrator or O_2 cylinder.

Examine each of the outward features of the O_2 concentrator or cylinder with the patient and family. Note each light, knob, or attachment that can be seen on the front or back of the device. Explain the purpose of the warning lights and alarms, and trigger them if possible. Have the patient or a family member turn on the concentrator or cylinder. Demonstrate the procedure for removing filters and other items on the equipment. Explain the frequency with which to clean and replace all filters, humidifiers, and tubing. The purpose of the monthly visit from the staff of the home-care company is to ensure proper operation of the O_2 equipment. Ask the patient and family questions about the material just discussed, and clarify and reexplain any points if necessary. Explain the procedure that will be followed each time a visit to the home is made.

Explain the purpose and operation of the back-up O_2 cylinder, and point out that it is intended to be used only in an emergency. It may be helpful to attach a piece of paper to the cylinder containing information on operation of the cylinder because the patient

PROCEDURES FOR SAFE STORAGE AND HANDLING OF CYLINDERS
IN THE FACILITIES OF A HOME-CARE COMPANY

1. Cylinders should be placed in a clearly designated and identified location. No-smoking signs should be displayed clearly.
2. Cylinders must be secured at all times.
   a. Large cylinders (M, G, H, and K sizes) should be secured to a wall with a heavy metal chain.
   b. Small cylinders (D and E sizes) should be kept in a rack constructed for the purpose of holding cylinders.
   c. Empty cylinders should be labeled clearly as "empty" and stored in a separate place from any full or partially full cylinders.
3. Any large cylinder containing less than 500 psig when returned to the warehouse should be considered empty and stored accordingly.
4. Any small cylinder containing less than 1000 psig should be considered empty and stored accordingly. (E cylinders may be used for short-transport situations *only*. When in doubt consider the partial cylinder empty and obtain a full cylinder.)
5. For partially full cylinders the pressure in the cylinder, the date of the reading, and the name of the person making the pressure reading should be marked clearly on the cylinder.
6. Storage facilities for cylinders should be well ventilated, clean, dry, and free of clutter.
   a. Cylinders should be kept away from any source of heat or sparks, such as compressors, exterior metal walls, radiators, and steam pipes.
   b. Compressed gases should never be exposed to temperatures >125° F.
7. When not in use, large cylinders should always have the caps in place. Small cylinders should have a dust cap or tape with an O ring in place.
8. Before any cylinder is used, the shoulder markings and the condition of the cylinder should be checked.
   a. No cylinder should be used if the last inspection date was 10 or more years ago.
   b. No cylinder should be used if the contents, manufacturer, and warnings on the label are not legible.
   c. No cylinder should be used if it is not clean and clearly labeled and if it has not been painted somewhat recently.
9. When cylinders are moved, they should be strapped securely to a cylinder cart and then pushed to the desired location.
10. Empty cylinders should have the valves completely closed and the caps in place at all times.
11. A cylinder wrench should be the only type of wrench used for regulator attachment.
    a. Do not use an adjustable wrench or pipe wrench.
    b. Do not use a vise-grip wrench or channel-lock pliers.
12. Cylinder carts, stands, no-smoking signs, wrenches, regulators, and cylinders should be placed in specific locations.

and family may not remember when the time comes to use the back-up cylinder. Demonstrate how to turn on the cylinder, connect tubing to the regulator, etc. Explain the significance of the gauges and point out the 500 psig level at which the home-care company is to be notified to replace the cylinder. Give the family a written explanation and example of how to determine the length of time a cylinder will last before it must be replaced.

If the patient will have an E cylinder for ambulation or travel, explain its operation and point out similarities and differences between the large and small cylinders. Explain that the pressure in the two cylinders is the same but that the amount of gas in each is very different. Discuss the valves, regulator, color of the cylinders, their labels, and the material they are made of. Demonstrate the way to use the cylinder cart, attachment of the regulator, and connection of tubing. Demonstrate how to turn on the cylinder, check the pressure in the cylinder, attach the tubing, and set the flow rate. Also have the patient and family move the cylinder (push it and pull it) around the room, down halls, and even outside the home if possible.

Review the written operating instructions for the O_2 concentrator, cylinders, and other devices. Provide the family with a checklist of the items to examine when checking the operation of the equipment (see Appendix C). Review emergency procedures and phone numbers if necessary. After completing this review and answering questions, have the patient and family sign a form that lists the items covered during the review. This form can serve as a record that all points have been covered and that the health-care provider installing the equipment did everything that was required. It can also serve as a receipt for the equipment. Unanswered questions and points needing clarification or follow-up can be noted. This form can then go to the director of patient services for the home-care company, and appropriate follow-up can be initiated.

Before leaving the home, thank the patient and anyone else present for their cooperation, and compliment them when it is appropriate. Assure them that someone will contact them shortly to review use of the equipment again and that someone from the home-care company is available 24 hours a day.

First impressions are important. All staff of the home-care company should be professional, courteous, and confident. Any staff member who is unsure of the answer to a question that a patient asks should not guess at the answer. Explain that you will find out the answer, then make sure you do. It may be best to remember that as a staff member from the home-care company, you are a foreigner and are invading the patient and family's home, their personal space. Do not be presumptuous, request permission before doing anything in their home, and be ready to accept "no" for an answer.

It is important that the patient and family try to perform each skill that is expected of them while they are being instructed and do not just watch. Remember from Chapter 3 to demonstrate, do, and then practice. The patient and family should remove and replace the filter, check the security of the humidifier and O_2 tubing,

ITEMS TO CHECK FOR PROPER FUNCTION OF O_2 THERAPY EQUIPMENT

Check that all alarms are operating.
Place control knob at various flow rates, and measure for accuracy at the patient's end of the tubing.
Check filter placement and cleanliness.
Check all tubing connections and the humidifier for secure attachment
Fill the humidifier with clean tap water or distilled water when available.
Change any soiled tubing or patient connecting devices.
Set flow rate on the prescribed setting, and inform the patient or other person present of the setting.

connect extra lengths of tubing, and fill the humidifier with water. They should be able to explain the significance of each warning light and the action to be taken when each light is on. Finally, they should post the telephone numbers for the physician and the ambulance service and the 24-hour telephone number for the home-care company near their telephone. This initial instruction means a lot of information being given in a short period of time. Assure the patient and family that help is as close as the telephone. A follow-up contact by a respiratory-care practitioner should be scheduled for 48 to 72 hours after the initial instruction. This follow-up can be done efficiently by phone but may at times require a personal visit.

Information needed by the home-care company

The physician is the primary source of information about the patient and the patient's O_2 prescription. The boxes on p. 179 list the information that should be supplied to the home-care company about the patient and the prescription from the physician. With this information the prescription can be correctly and thoroughly implemented, and requests for reimbursement from third-party payers can be expedited.

If patient discharge is imminent, a delivery person with the home-care company should be contacted immediately. This person should be given the patient's name, address, and telephone number and as much other information on the patient and the order as is available. A visit to the patient's home and assessment of the patient in the home should be completed within 24 hours of the installation of equipment and arrival of the patient at home. During this visit, particular attention should be given to any questions that arose from the instructions given during equipment installation.

COST OF O_2 THERAPY

When a physician prescribes O_2 for a patient, it can be supplied by almost any home-care company and by some pharmacies. One question that should be considered

INFORMATION TO BE OBTAINED ABOUT THE PATIENT

Name
Present address
Location where equipment is to be placed, including address (with county)
Names of spouse, relatives, or friends
Home and work telephone numbers for the patient and spouse or relative
County health care number, if applicable
Medicare number, if applicable
Medicaid number, if applicable
Name of private insurance company, if applicable
Patient's account number with private insurance company
Name of referral source (ordering physician)
Address of referral source
Telephone number of referral source
Name of discharging hospital
Address of discharging hospital
Telephone number of discharging hospital
Name of person giving patient information
Date and time order received

CLINICAL AND PRESCRIPTION INFORMATION
NEEDED FROM THE PHYSICIAN

Date and time of expected discharge from the hospital
Diagnosis
Pa_{O_2} value at rest and during exercise
Prescription to be administered
Number of liters per minute at rest and during activity
Number of hours per day of use
Device ordered (for example, concentrator, cylinders, or O_2 cannula)
Does the patient require O_2 for travel?
Is the patient ambulatory? Is ambulation restricted to the home, or can the patient also
    move around outside the home?
Is exercise prescribed? What type of activity? Any limits? How often? What O_2 flow rate
    is prescribed during the activity?*
If O_2 is not continuous, how many hours per day should it be used?†

*If O_2 is prescribed with activities or exercise, flow rate should be approximately 1 to 2 L/min greater than at rest. Maintain O_2 saturation >85%.
†If nocturnal O_2 is ordered, it should be administered for at least 18 hours per day.

when using O_2 is who will pay for it. If the physician prescribes O_2 and the patient is willing to pay for it, obtaining O_2 is no different from going to the pharmacy to have any other prescription filled. O_2 use in the home can be expensive. Often the patient is covered by a medical-insurance program, and the insurance company has established criteria detailing when it will pay for O_2 and when it will not. This discrepancy makes acquiring O_2 for home use a more complex issue than acquiring most other prescription drugs. The wide variety of delivery systems also contributes to the complexity of home O_2 therapy. Training in equipment operation and follow-up on the condition of the patient and the performance of equipment are important. The system must fit the lifestyle and rehabilitation goals of the patient. Home-care companies assist the physician and the patient in selecting the most appropriate O_2 system to use and in working through the bureaucracies involved in medical reimbursement.

Most insurance companies follow the guidelines recommended by Medicare for reimbursement of charges for O_2 therapy. A Pao_2 of less than 55 mm Hg and a pulse oximetry value of O_2 saturation less than 85% are beginning to be accepted by many insurance companies and by Medicare. Patients with an arterial Pao_2 >55 mm Hg at rest that falls below this value during exertion can also be reimbursed for the cost of O_2 therapy. In the latter case the O_2 used during exertion is the only O_2 that will be covered by the insurance company. To document this decrease in Pao_2, it may be necessary to obtain a measure of arterial O_2 during an activity, such as walking (see Chapter 5, a desaturation index and an occupational study).

Third-party reimbursement

Third-party reimbursement for medical care is a complex issue. Hundreds of billions of dollars a year in medical costs are paid not by the individual receiving the service but by private, state, or federal insurance programs. Reimbursement for services and equipment involved in pulmonary rehabilitation and home care has not been supported well by the insurance system. In 1965 federal legislation was written establishing the Medicare and Medicaid programs under the Social Security Act. In this legislation no provision was made for respiratory care or pulmonary rehabilitation. This omission has led to continuing problems in providing quality respiratory care in the home to the pulmonary patient. The legislation also established the Health Care Finance Administration (HCFA) under the U.S. Department of Health and Human Services (at that time the Department of Health, Education, and Welfare). The HCFA has the responsibility of administering the Medicare and Medicaid programs and other health-insurance programs at the federal level.

HCFA interprets legislation written by Congress, establishes regulations needed to implement this legislation, and supervises adherence to these regulations. The states are grouped by HCFA into regions, each with its own administration that interprets and implements the national regulations. Each of the states that make up a region uses a local health-insurance company to act as the carrier, or administrator, for Medicare in that state. The carrier's responsibility is to implement the regulations established by the regional HCFA, to provide payment when these regulations are met, and to reject reimbursement when the regulations are not met. Making these choices gives the local carrier a great deal of power and responsibility. This carrier is different in each state, and a large state may even have more than one carrier for different areas of the state. One part of Medicare may be administered by one insurance carrier, and another part may be administered by a separate carrier. Other federal programs of health insurance such as the railroad retirement, military retirement, and mine workers' programs, have separate carriers within each state. The increasing complexity involved in interpreting regulations as they filter down from the federal level has allowed for not only flexibility but also variation in the interpretation of the regulations from region to region of the country.

Medicare

Medicare is divided into two parts. Part A includes reimbursement for health care in the hospital or skilled nursing facility. Part B includes reimbursement for health services through home-care and DME companies. Types of home-care services covered under Medicare, Part B include nursing services, physical therapy, and other therapies specifically mentioned in the Social Security Act. Payment for respiratory-therapy equipment in the home has been included under the guidelines of Medicare, Part B that address DME. Since respiratory care is not mentioned in the Social Security Act, there has been no provision for coverage of respiratory-care services, only for respiratory-therapy equipment used in the home.

In each state, implementation of Medicare regulations rests with a different insurance carrier. Because each carrier can implement the regulations according to its own interpretation, the cost of items or services that would be reimbursable under Medicare in one state may not be reimbursable in a neighboring state. For example, consider the situation in which a patient with a pulmonary disease was confined temporarily to a wheelchair, before which the patient had been prescribed O_2 at 2 L/min when walking and 1 L/min at rest. When the patient was confined to the wheelchair and used it as the primary means of mobility, Medicare refused to cover the cost of the additional O_2 required for ambulation because it was decided that ambulation consisted of walking and not moving around in a wheelchair.

It would be helpful if the patient were to understand somewhat how the criteria are established for reimbursement of services or equipment in the home. HCFA receives input from its regions and state carriers for suggested reimbursement guidelines. Requests are made by HCFA for comments on proposed regulations in the Federal Register. After these comments are received by HCFA and hearings on the regulations are held, policy statements on reimbursement are published as "final notice" in the

Federal Register. These new regulations are also disseminated to the individual carriers in each state to be implemented in that state. Generally these regulations specify requirements that must be met before the cost of services or equipment is reimbursed (see the section on reimbursement for O_2 therapy in the home, beginning on p. 178). If reimbursement is denied by the carrier, an appeal may be made to the carrier and ultimately to HCFA in what is called a "fair hearing." At this hearing the people involved, such as physicians, patient representatives, and hospital personnel, meet with the carrier to discuss specific arguments to justify the requested reimbursement.

DME use in the home involves a wide assortment of equipment that can be purchased or rented for the patient through Medicare. Although the cost of aerosol-therapy equipment, suction devices, and some other therapeutic equipment is reimbursed through Medicare, the respiratory-care item costing the most to Medicare is O_2. In the early 1980s the General Accounting Office (GAO) of the federal government reviewed payment practices for DME under Medicare. The subsequent report showed that reimbursement policies should be made more consistent throughout the country. Criteria established in the regulations could have been followed very strictly in one state and very loosely in another state. After years of soliciting comments and holding hearings, HCFA announced a new policy concerning the use of O_2 and O_2 equipment in the home, which went into effect September 1, 1985. This new policy represents major changes in reimbursement of the cost of O_2 therapy.

Medicaid is a separate federal program for providing health-care coverage to those who do not meet Medicare requirements and cannot supply their own insurance. The program is administered through each state with federal funds being given to each state according to the services provided. The greatest difference between Medicaid and Medicare is that Medicaid pays only 80% of a certain allowable amount, which is based on the most common charges for that service within the state. Also the service must be approved by Medicaid before it is performed to qualify for reimbursement.

COVERAGE OF O_2 THERAPY IN THE HOME

The most recent policy for reimbursement in O_2 therapy in the home is found in the Federal Register.* The following summary of this policy statement outlines the criteria for Medicare coverage of O_2 services provided in the home. The policy is often also used by other third-party insurance carriers as their policy for reimbursement of home O_2 use.

Medical documentation

The physician writing the prescription for O_2 use must include in it the following items to qualify for reimbursement:

Diagnosis of the disease requiring home O_2 use

---

*Federal Register 50(66):13,742-13,750, April 5, 1985.

Flow rate and O_2 concentration

"Estimate" of the frequency and duration of use

If the patient's condition improves or deteriorates causing a change in the need for O_2, the physician will need to provide new documentation for a revised prescription. A review of medical necessity should be done every 6 to 12 months, depending on the patient's condition and regional Medicare requirements. This review may at times be done by telephone, or it may require an ABG sample or ear/pulse oximetry.

Laboratory evidence

The initial claim to the Medicare carrier must include the *results* of a study to determine the Po_2 in the blood. A measurement may be made of arterial Po_2 *or* arterial O_2 saturation through ear/pulse oximetry. The conditions under which the study was conducted (such as with the patient at rest, sleeping, exercising, on room air, or on O_2) must be stated. The patient's body position during the test and any other information that would affect interpretation of the test results should also be included.

Conditions for coverage of home O_2 therapy

Coverage of home O_2 therapy is provided for patients with *significant hypoxemia in a chronic, stable state*, for example, severe lung disease, such as COPD, diffuse interstitial lung disease, cystic fibrosis, bronchiectasis, or pulmonary neoplasm. A second major area of coverage for O_2 therapy is *hypoxia-related symptoms* that may improve with O_2 therapy. Some of these symptoms are pulmonary hypertension, erythrocytosis, impairment of cognitive processes, nocturnal restlessness, morning headache, and CHF caused by cor pulmonale.

Evidence of significant hypoxia must be demonstrated by an *arterial Po_2 at or below 55 mm Hg or an arterial O_2 saturation at or below 85% when measured at rest and breathing room air.* An arterial Po_2 at or below 55 mm Hg or an arterial O_2 saturation at or below 85% during sleep for a patient who demonstrates a Po_2 above 55 mm Hg or an arterial O_2 saturation at 85% while awake will also be accepted.

Coverage may also be granted for O_2 therapy in circumstances in which the O_2 level falls more than normal during sleep, for example, a decrease in arterial Po_2 of more than 10 mm Hg or a decrease in arterial O_2 saturation of more than 5%. In cases in which desaturation, or a fall in Po_2, is noted during sleep but not during waking periods, O_2 therapy will be covered only for nocturnal use. For the patient who has an arterial Po_2 greater than 56 mm Hg or an arterial O_2 saturation greater than 86% at rest and breathing room air and whose Po_2 has fallen below 55 mm Hg and arterial O_2 saturation has fallen below 85% during exercise, O_2 therapy will be covered only during exercise.

Coverage for O_2 therapy in the home may be provided for patients whose arterial Po_2 falls between 56 and 59 mm Hg or whose arterial O_2 saturation is between 86% and 89% if any of the following conditions is present:

CHF with edema

A P-wave greater than 3 ml in the standard lead II, 3 or AVF ("P" pulmonale on
   the electrocardiogram [ECG])
A hematocrit greater than 56%
Patients whose arterial Po_2 is greater than 60 mm Hg and whose arterial O_2
saturation is greater than 90% will have home O_2 therapy presumed not medically
necessary. This presumption can be disputed with the insurance carrier, and appropri-
ate documentation can be provided to justify reimbursement of its cost. Coverage for
the cost of O_2 therapy will not be provided for the following conditions:
   Angina pectoris in the absence of hypoxemia
   Breathlessness without evidence of cor pulmonale or hypoxemia
   Severe peripheral vascular disease
   Terminal illnesses not affecting the lungs

Portable O_2 systems

Portable O_2 systems are now covered by Medicare as complementary to a stationary system or by themselves for intermittent use, such as during exercise. The medical
documentation included in the request for reimbursement should describe the activities and exercise routines that the patient is to perform on a regular basis. This
description should include a medically therapeutic purpose for a portable system that
cannot be met by a stationary system. The documentation should include a statement
that use of the portable O_2 system during activity or exercise improves the patient's
clinical situation. This improvement may be demonstrated by the patient's ability to
exercise and perform various activities with O_2 that could not have been performed
without O_2.

BIBLIOGRAPHY

Bell W et al: Home care and rehabilitation in respiratory medicine, Philadelphia, 1984, JB Lippincott Co.
Compressed Gas Association, Inc: Oxygen (pamphlet G-4), Arlington, Va, 1980.
Hodgkin JE, Zorn E, and Connors G: Pulmonary rehabilitation: guidelines to success, Stoneham, Mass,
   1984, Butterworth Publishers.
Medicare program: Coverage of oxygen for use in a patient's home, Federal Register 50(66):13,742-13,750,
   1985.
O'Ryan JA and Burns DG: Pulmonary rehabilitation: from hospital to home, Chicago, 1984, Year Book
   Medical Publishers, Inc.
Wenmark WH: Suggested guidelines for respiratory therapy home care, revised 1978, American Association
   for Respiratory Therapy: Committee on Rehabilitation and Continuing Care.
Young DA: Quality care for the chronic lung disease patient living at home, Am Lung Assoc Bull 2-6, Dec/
   Jan 1978.

Interviewing the patient and family

SUGGESTED QUESTIONS TO USE DURING AN INTERVIEW WITH A PATIENT WITH A PULMONARY DISORDER

The following questionnaire is useful for obtaining the information described in the list of topics in Chapter 2. Through use of this questionnaire, the pulmonary disorder can be identified, symptoms can be cataloged, and complaints can be clarified. These questions are intended to serve as a guide during the interview process. They should not be used exactly as written but should be adapted to the situation.

IDENTIFYING THE PRIMARY COMPLAINT

Why are you seeking medical care?
What symptoms prompted you to act at this time?
When did you last feel well?
When did symptoms begin?

Symptoms (complaints) should be cataloged in order of onset. Each symptom should be described in terms of the following areas:
   Acute—onset within the past few days
   Subacute—onset more than a few days or weeks ago and duration of more than a few days or weeks
   Chronic—onset more than several months ago and duration of more than several months
   Stationary or progressing—change from past symptoms
   Complications and exacerbations

DETAILS OF SYMPTOMS AND COMPLAINTS
Cough

How often do you have a cough?
When do you usually cough (for example, when rising in the morning)?

Adapted from American College of Chest Physicians—American Thoracic Society modified pulmonary questionnaire.

Do you usually cough during the rest of the day or night?
    How often do you cough during the day or night?
How many times a day and how many days a week do you cough (for example, 4 or
    more times a day and 4 or more days a week)?
For how many consecutive months over how many years have you had a cough (for
    example, 3 or more consecutive months for 2 or more years)?
For how many years have you had this cough?
During which months does your cough give you the most trouble?
Have there been any changes in your cough recently?

Sputum production

Does your cough usually produce mucus?
At what time of day is your cough most productive?
Do you bring up phlegm during the rest of the day or night?
How often do you usually bring up phlegm (for example, two or more times a day)?
    How many days a week?
Have you brought up phlegm this frequently most days for 3 or more consecutive
    months during the year?
For how many years have you had trouble with phlegm production? .
During what times of year do you have more (or less) trouble with phlegm production?
What is the usual color of the phlegm you produce?
Does the color of your mucus change? How often? When? To what color does it
    change?

Episodes of cough and sputum production

Have you had periods or episodes of (increased) cough and sputum production lasting
    for 3 or more consecutive weeks in a year?
For how long does one of these episodes last?
For how many years have you had at least one such episode per year?
Do you awaken at night with a cough? How often each week? How often each night?

Wheezing

Do you ever hear a wheezing or whistling sound in your chest when you breathe?
How frequently does this occur?
When does this occur (for example, when you have a chest cold or head cold)?
How often does this occur when you do not have a cold?
Is it more likely to occur at night or during the day?
For how many years has this wheezing been occurring?
Have you ever had an attack of wheezing that has made you feel short of breath?
Have you had two or more such attacks?
How old were you when you first had such an attack?

Have you ever required medicine or other treatment for these wheezing episodes? What was this medicine? What did this treatment consist of?

Are you currently receiving medicine or other treatment for wheezing? What is this medicine? What does this treatment consist of?

Are there any particular months during which the wheezing episodes get worse or better? What are these months?

Shortness of breath

Are you ever troubled by shortness of breath when walking?

Are you ever troubled by shortness of breath during restful activities?

Are you troubled by shortness of breath when walking quickly on level ground or walking up a slight hill?

Does SOB cause you to have to walk more slowly than people your own age when on level ground because of shortness of breath?

Do you ever have to stop for breath when walking at your own pace on level ground?

Do you ever have to stop for breath after walking at your own pace for approximately 100 yards or after walking a few minutes on level ground?

Are you too short of breath to leave the house, or do you become short of breath when dressing and undressing?

For how long have you been experiencing shortness of breath at these times?

Are there any months when the episodes of shortness of breath are worse or better?

Do you ever awaken at night with shortness of breath? How often each week does this occur? How many times each night?

Chest colds and other chest illnesses

If you get a cold, does it usually go to your chest?

When you have a chest cold, does it usually clear up within a week, or does it seem to give you more trouble than it gives most people?

During the past 3 years, have you had any chest illnesses that have kept you off work, at home indoors, or in bed?

Did you see a physician for this illness? What was the diagnosis?

What treatment was prescribed? How well did the treatment relieve your symptoms?

OTHER TOPICS FOR DISCUSSION DURING THE INTERVIEW
Past illnesses

Did you have any lung trouble before the age of 16? If so, please describe it.

Have you ever had an attack of bronchitis confirmed by a doctor? At what age was your first attack? At what other times have they occurred?

Have you ever had pneumonia confirmed by a doctor? When did you have it? How often have you had it?

Have you ever been diagnosed by a doctor as having chronic bronchitis? Is it still being treated? At what age did symptoms begin to occur, and at what age was the condition diagnosed?

Have you ever had emphysema diagnosed by a physician? Is it still being treated? At what age did symptoms begin to occur? At what age was it diagnosed?

Have you ever had asthma diagnosed by a doctor? Do you currently require medicine or other treatment for your asthma? At what age did it start? At what age did it stop? Was it ever associated with allergies?

Have you ever had hay fever, respiratory allergies, or sensitivity to cold air? Do you still have any of these problems? At what age did it start? What type of medical treatment did you receive for the condition?

Have you ever had sinus trouble or nasal polyps? Have you ever had your tonsils removed?

Have you ever had any other chest diseases, such as bronchiectasis, tuberculosis, cancer, or an occupational disease? What treatment did you receive? When did you receive treatment?

Have you ever had any chest operations or chest injuries? If so, please explain.

Have you ever smoked cigarettes? Do you presently smoke?

How old were you when you started to smoke cigarettes regularly?

If you have stopped smoking cigarettes, how old were you when you stopped?

How many cigarettes do you smoke per day now?

On the average, of the entire time you smoked, how many cigarettes did you smoke per day? (Calculate pack years [Packs per day × Number of years])

Have you ever smoked a pipe regularly?

How old were you when you started to smoke a pipe regularly?

Do you inhale the pipe smoke? Did you inhale it in the past?

Have you ever smoked cigars regularly?

How old were you when you started to smoke cigars regularly?

Do you inhale the cigar smoke? Did you inhale it in the past?

Have you ever lived with a person who smoked around you regularly? What did this person smoke? For how long each day were you exposed to this smoke? For how many years were you exposed to it?

Occupational history

Record occupational history chronologically from early adulthood to the present.

What types of jobs have you held?

Name of company

Location: geographic location of company as related to location of home, assigned space in the work place, and tasks involved

Duration of employment, changes in position

Illnesses or injuries on the job, job-related or otherwise

Assessment of physical and emotional/psychologic stress

Protective equipment used on the job

Potential relationships between the present condition and past occupational exposure:

Chronic bronchitis—Smoke, dust, and fumes

Silicosis—Mining

Emphysema—Environment and smoking at work

Berylliosis—Manufacturing light bulbs

Byssinosis—Manufacturing using cotton

Interstitial pneumonia—Farm work involving silos

Histoplasmosis—Chicken dung

Asthma—Farming and grain dust

Asbestosis—Mining and contact with insulation

Have you ever worked for a year or more at a dusty job? For how many years did you work there?

What type of dust was present?

Was the dust exposure mild, moderate, or severe?

Have you ever been exposed to gas or chemical fumes in the work place? What type of gas or fumes? For how many years were you exposed?

Was the gas exposure mild, moderate, or severe?

At what occupation have you worked longest?

Family history

Have there been any serious illnesses, especially those causing death, in the immediate family? Have grandparents, aunts, or uncles had such diseases?

Is there any hereditary predisposition to a pulmonary disorder, including any of the following?

α_1 antitrypsin deficiency or emphysema

Cystic fibrosis

Asthma, childhood and/or adult, with exercise

Tuberculosis or other infectious disease

What type of illnesses and treatments have you had in the past? How severe have the illnesses been?

Have you had infectious diseases of childhood, pneumonia, and prolonged or complicated illnesses?

Have you had injuries or operations?

Have you had dental extraction or surgery?

What medical treatment have you received for illness?

Treatments received

Response to therapy, anesthesia, or surgery

Complications encountered

Was either of your natural parents ever diagnosed as having any of the following chronic lung conditions: chronic bronchitis, emphysema, asthma, or lung cancer?

Is this parent currently living? What is the age and condition of this parent?

Do any members of your family other than your parents have any of the lung problems mentioned? Have they had them in the past?

Has your doctor ever told you that you have heart trouble? What was the problem, and how is it being treated?

Have you had heart trouble in the past 10 years? What was the problem, and how was it treated?

Has a doctor ever told you that you have high blood pressure? When was it identified, and how is it being treated?

Have you ever had surgery? What type of surgery was it? What type of anesthesia was used?

Have you ever had any problems with your lungs after surgery?

Do you have any other questions about your lungs or breathing that I have not asked?

Personal history

Record personal history, especially as it relates to disabilities.

Background, living habits, and environment

List chronologically places of residence and lengths of stay for living and travel experiences. Special note should be made of the following conditions and the areas in which they are prominent:

Histoplasmosis—Areas around the Ohio, Mississippi, and St. Lawrence rivers

Coccidioidomycosis—Desert areas and the southwestern United States

Schistosomiasis—Puerto Rico, Central America, and Egypt

Establish past and present socioeconomic status from the patient's perspective.

Evidence of malnutrition

Poor hygiene, water quality, and sanitary conditions

Past and present abuse of tobacco, marijuana, or other substances

Length of time as a smoker

Type of devices (filtered or unfiltered) used

If you have quit, how long ago was it? Why did you quit?

Amount used per day

Number of pack years

Allergies, established or suspected, including allergies to animals, pets, flowers, plants, and other allergens

Patient and family education

Following is suggested content for a patient-education program in COPD. Topics are broken down to give more detail, which may be included in the material presented to the patient and family. Not all material should be covered with every patient. Only the material that is relevant to a patient's individual situation should be covered with that patient.

GENERAL EDUCATION

Anatomy and physiology of the cardiopulmonary system
    Upper and lower respiratory tract
    How each tract works and the role each one plays in protecting the lungs
    Process of gas exchange and respiration
    Cardiopulmonary circulation, blood pressure in the lungs and the rest of the body, pulse, and respiratory rate
    Gross anatomy of the upper and lower airway
        Function of the nose
        Function of the larynx in swallowing
        Function of mucus and the mucociliary escalator
        Exchange of O_2 and CO_2 in the alveoli
        Relationship between the heart and lungs
        Muscles of respiration and their action
COPD—Pathophysiology, diagnostic tests, and contributing factors
    The nature of emphysema, chronic bronchitis, asthma, bronchiectasis, and cor pulmonale
    Effects on health of smoking, occupational exposure, air pollution, allergies, hereditary factors, and infection
    The chest roentgenogram, pulmonary-function tests, blood-gas assays, and bronchoscopy
Manifestations of COPD—symptoms and progression
    Early symptoms of chronic lung disease: SOB, sputum, wheezing, and cough
    Later symptoms: fatigue, weight loss, changes in sleep habits, edema, psychologic changes, and cyanosis
    Specific pathophysiology of the disease
    Specific symptoms of the disease experienced by the patient

Effects of inactivity
Medical terminology and symbols
  Pulmonary terminology
  Definition of diseases, anatomy terms, and physiology terms
  Explanation of symbols commonly used in medicine
  Explanation of the medical-records system
Roles and responsibilities of team members
  Create a list of all the roles of people who will be in contact with the patient or family.
  Provide names of people in these roles.
  List contact persons for given situations and ways to contact them.
  Discuss who is ultimately responsible for the patient's care.
    Responsibilities of the physician
    Responsibilities of the patient
    Responsibilities of family members
    Responsibilities of therapists, nurses, and social workers
    Responsibilities of the DME company
  Discuss the reasons for certain persons' coming to see the patient.
  Discuss what each person will be doing during the visit, how often each person will visit, and when these visits will take place.
Warning signs and patient evaluation
  Establishing baseline data through characterization of symptoms: wheezing, SOB, exercise intolerance, sputum production, an unclear sensorium, change in appetite, change in sleep habits, and edema
  Identifying personal irritants
  Identifying a significant change in the patient's condition
  Recording results from the patient examination and maintaining the patient's record
  Knowing whom to notify with findings from a patient assessment
  Recognizing an emergency
  Recognizing an infection and when to take antibiotics
  Administering flu vaccines and instructing the patient to avoid infection and second-hand smoke

INDIVIDUALIZED INSTRUCTION

Medications and other therapeutic treatments
  General information: action, name, and dosage of the drug, schedule for administration, possible side effects, and drug interactions; use and abuse of over-the-counter medications; special precautions; operation and cleaning of equipment; preparation of medications, safety of medication use, and prescription for O_2

Nutrition and hydration
    Composition of a balanced diet, how and when to eat, problem foods and special
        diets, adequate fluid intake (quantity and quality)
    Dietary needs and special diets
    Tube feeding
    Special methods of food preparation
Smoking cessation
    Community resources for help
    Nature of the habit
    Various helpful techniques for quitting
ADL and energy conservation
    Work-efficiency principle, counseling in performance of leisure and household
        activities and personal-hygiene activities
    Energy-conservation measures and planning
Breathing retraining and breathing exercises
    Diaphragmatic and pursed-lip breathing techniques, control of breathing under
        stress and with work, control of cough, ventilation retraining with ADL,
        modified calisthenics, segmental breathing, posture, motion and breathing,
        and orthopnea
Operation, care, and cleaning of respiratory equipment
    Large- and small-reservoir nebulizers, O_2 humidifiers, room humidifiers, O_2
        equipment, and suction devices
Administration of therapeutic treatments
    Aerosol therapy, bronchial drainage, percussion/vibration, using an MDI, breath-
        ing patterns with aerosols
Strength and endurance training
    Graded physical exercise, building strength and endurance, safety, prescription,
        and maintaining physical activity
Relaxation training
    Jacobsen's technique, meditation, imagery, why and when to perform training,
        biofeedback, and yoga
Community resources for COPD patients
    Social services, lung association, recreational resources, maid or meal service,
        emergency facilities, and home health-care companies
Record keeping and personal health care
    Daily diary of activities, symptoms, medications, and meals
    Case history, test results, and diagnosis on hand
Insurance and third-party reimbursement
    Medicare and Medicaid and private insurance
    Social Security
    Insurance forms
Psychologic aspects of disability

Family relationships, motivators, hobbies, communication skills, lost self-esteem, social outlets, panic, stress in the work place, travel, and sexual activity

MECHANICAL VENTILATION

Ventilation and the mechanical ventilator
    Operation of the ventilator—what it does and how it performs
    Power source—locations and types
    Controls on the ventilator—the effects of each one
    Monitoring systems, gauges, and alarms
    Procedure to follow if an alarm sounds or a gauge indicates a problem
    Maintenance of the ventilator and patient circuit
    Changing the patient ventilator circuit
    Cleaning the ventilator and circuit
    Completing the ventilator flow sheet
    Trouble-shooting the ventilator, for example, for leaks
    Procedure to follow during a power failure or other emergency
    Humidification system
Manual-resuscitation bag
    Assembly and disassembly of the bag
    Connection of the bag to the patient
    Operation of the bag
    Cleaning of the bag
    Naming each part of the bag
Suctioning procedure and tracheostomy care
    Equipment required
    Operation of equipment
    Trouble-shooting of equipment
    Procedure for suctioning or tracheostomy care
    Irrigation procedures
    Preoxygenation, reoxygenation, and hyperinflation
    Stoma care
    Tracheostomy-tube cleaning
    Changing dressings and ties
    Changing the tracheostomy tube
    Operation of the cuff
    Determining when to suction
    Frequency of tracheostomy care
Emergency procedures
    Cardiopulmonary resuscitation (CPR)
    Reinsertion of the artificial airway

Calling emergency contacts and services
Other airway problems
Power failure
Equipment malfunction

MISCELLANEOUS

General nursing-care needs
Moving the patient in the bed and positioning the patient
Making the patient's bed
Skin care, especially with a curass
Examining the stoma for infection
Mouth care and dental hygiene
Daily personal hygiene
Use of a bedpan or bedside commode
Exercises in bed
Weighing the patient
Control of the home environment
Control of temperature, humidity, and dust
Cleaning of systems and changing of filters
Spatial requirements for equipment
Opportunities for patient mobility
Psychosocial aspects of patient care and family needs
Diversionary activities for the patient and family
Communication with the patient
Visitors
Trips and outside activities
Hobbies
Other needs, medical or otherwise
Accessing community resources
Insurance requirements
Payment for home-care services
Ordering supplies
Emergency services and phone numbers
Notification of utility companies
Preparation of normal saline and distilled water solutions for home use

Forms for use in home care

C-1, DAILY DIARY

Name: _____ Date: _____

Use one form for each day. Write down anything about your activities and your condition during the day. How do you feel? How does your breathing feel? What are you doing during the day? What difficulties and questions have you encountered? These items can be discussed with your physician or the rehabilitation-program staff during your next visit. Bring these records along to your visit so that any patterns can be noted by the health-care practitioners. Use another sheet of paper if you need more room, but be sure to note the time.

Time	Comments
6 to 8 AM	_____
8 to 9 AM	_____
9 to 10 AM	_____
10 to 11 AM	_____
11 AM to 12 PM	_____
12 to 1 PM	_____
1 to 2 PM	_____
2 to 3 PM	_____
3 to 4 PM	_____
4 to 5 PM	_____
5 to 6 PM	_____
6 to 7 PM	_____
7 to 8 PM	_____
8 to 9 PM	_____
9 PM to 12 AM	_____

General comments (any points to bring up for discussion at your next visit):

C-2, EXERCISE CHECK-OFF SHEET

Name: _____

For the period: _____ to _____

Activities and exercises that are part of your present program are listed below. They will change as your needs change and as you learn new exercises. The number of times or length of time an activity is to be performed is also given. *Do not go too fast.* See Appendix G for a description of the activity.

Day of the week
Place a check mark on the line when the activity has been completed.

Activity	Mon.	Tues.	Wed.	Thurs.	Fri.	Sat.	Sun.
Diaphragmatic breathing with pursed lips for 10 minutes	___	___	___	___	___	___	___
Forward bends or side bends for 10 minutes three times each week	___	___	___	___	___	___	___
Knee bends or toe raises for 10 minutes three times each week	___	___	___	___	___	___	___
Arm circles or arm raises for 10 minutes three times each week	___	___	___	___	___	___	___
Scissor kicks or leg lifts for 10 minutes three times each week	___	___	___	___	___	___	___
Sit-ups or head raises for 10 minutes three times each week	___	___	___	___	___	___	___
Walking or stair climbing for 20 minutes four times each week	___	___	___	___	___	___	___
_____	___	___	___	___	___	___	___
_____	___	___	___	___	___	___	___
_____	___	___	___	___	___	___	___

C-3, YOUR SYMPTOM RECORD (GETTING TO KNOW YOURSELF)

Answer the following questions over the next week. Fill in the space or line with the information requested.

What is your pulse rate? Count for 15 seconds, and write the number on the line below. Do this in the morning before getting out of bed.

Mon. _____   Tues. _____   Wed. _____   Thurs. _____

Fri. _____.   Sat. _____   Sun. _____

What is your body temperature before getting out of bed? Use an oral thermometer, and wait 3 minutes before reading it. Write the number on the line below.

Mon. _____   Tues. _____   Wed. _____   Thurs. _____

Fri. _____   Sat. _____   Sun. _____

When do you experience an episode of SOB? Does it occur only when you are performing an activity? What is the activity? Do you feel SOB when you are *not* performing some activity? Mark the time(s) of day when you usually feel SOB.

6 to 9 AM [   ]   9 AM to 12 PM [   ]

12 to 3 PM [   ]   3 to 5 PM   [   ]   5 to 8 PM   [   ]

8 to 10 PM [   ]   10 PM to 12 AM [   ]

During the night, 12 to 6 AM   [   ]

_____

_____

How often each week do you experience episodes of SOB? When do these episodes occur? How do you deal with them?

All day, every day   [   ]   Several times each day   [   ]

Only when I am active   [   ]   Several days each week   [   ]

On which days have you experienced SOB this week? _____

_____

Every night   [ ]   Several nights each week   [ ]

At what time of night do they usually occur? _____

Other times or occasions when you experience SOB _____

_____

SPUTUM PRODUCTION

When you produce sputum, what is it like?

	When?	How much?	What color?	How thick?
Monday	_____	_____	_____	_____
Tuesday	_____	_____	_____	_____
Wednesday	_____	_____	_____	_____
Thursday	_____	_____	_____	_____
Friday	_____	_____	_____	_____
Saturday	_____	_____	_____	_____
Sunday	_____	_____	_____	_____

COUGH

When do you have a cough?

All day, every day   [ ]

Only in the morning   [ ]

At different times each day   [ ]   When: _____

Several times each week   [ ]   When: _____

Do you always produce sputum with a cough?   Yes [ ]   No [ ]

Is your cough usually "dry"?   Yes [ ]   No [ ]

OTHER SYMPTOMS

Do you ever notice swelling of ankles or fingers?   Yes [ ]   No [ ]

When: _____

Do you ever have headaches immediately after waking in the morning?

Yes [   ]   No [   ]

When: _____

Do you need to sleep on several pillows or sitting up?

Always [   ]   Never [   ]   Occasionally [   ]

When: _____

Do you ever experience any of the following?   Chest pain [   ]

Loss of appetite [   ]   Blood in sputum [   ]   Dizziness [   ]

A "racing" HR [   ]

When: _____

Is your breathing more difficult at certain times of the year?

When: Fall [   ]   Winter [   ]   Spring [   ]   Summer [   ]

Do you have allergies that affect your breathing?   Yes [   ]   No [   ]

What are they? _____

_____

_____

_____

_____

Daily record for home mechanical ventilation

Place a check mark in the box next to the items that have been checked. Place the appropriate number in the box for those items that are read, measured, or counted.

Date:

Time:

Percentage of O_2:

Breathing rate per minute—
  Of the ventilator:
  Of the patient:

Volume setting:

Ventilation mode:

Highest pressure:

Time to inhale:

Time to exhale:

Time to trigger the low-pressure alarm:

Highest inhaled flow-rate setting:

Water heater setting:

Inhaled pressure limit alarm setting:

Pressure in the O_2 cylinder:

Humidifier filled with water:

Low-pressure alarm working:

Manual ventilation bag operational:

Tracheostomy care done:

Ventilator circuit changed:

Aerosol treatment given:

Other:

Other:

Initials of the person doing the check or procedure:

Patient's name:

Appendix C-4

C-5, CHECK SHEET FOR EQUIPMENT INSTALLATION IN THE HOME

Examine or discuss each of the following items, and note your findings. Check each item when it has been assessed. Make any comments in the space provided. Include factors that may present a problem to the patient and/or the equipment. Keep in mind safety, convenience, and family lifestyle.

Comments

___ Entrances and exits to the home:

___ Location of heaters and registers:

___ Location and number of electrical outlets (grounding, circuit capacity):

___ Location of the patient's bed:

___ Location of a chair for the patient:

___ Location of the patient's commode (distance to the bathroom):

___ Accessibility of respiratory equipment:

___ Daily habits and lifestyle:

___ Location of windows in the patient's room:

___ Location of the patient's room (as related to the remainder of the house and the family):

___ Location of backup systems for equipment:

___ Location of cleaning and drying area for equipment:

___ Storage space for supplies:

___ Distance in the home to be walked or moved around in:

___ Disposal of supplies and waste
materials:

___ Obstacles or hazards for O_2 tubing:

___ Operation of equipment:

___ Cleaning of equipment:

___ Assembly of equipment:

___ Emergency procedures and numbers:

___ Prescription from physician:

Comments and other notes:

_____

_____

_____

_____

Signature of home health-care provider: _____

Date: _____

Signature of patient or family member: _____

Date: _____

C-6, LIST OF IMPORTANT PHONE NUMBERS, ADDRESSES, AND OTHER INFORMATION

Name of patient: _____

    Address: _____

_____

    Phone: (Home) _____ - _____ (Work) _____ - _____

Name of nearest relative: _____

    Address: _____

_____

    Phone: (Home) _____ - _____ (Work) _____ - _____

Name of nearby neighbor: _____

    Address: _____

_____

    Location of this neighbor's home in relation to your home:

_____

_____

    Phone: (Home) _____ - _____ (Work) _____ - _____

Name of primary-care physician: _____

    Address: _____

_____

    Phone: (Home) _____ - _____ (Work) _____ - _____

        Beeper (paging) number: _____ - _____

        Name of office nurse or assistant: _____

Name of pulmonary physician: _____

    Address: _____

    _____

    Phone: (Home) _____-_____ (Work) _____-_____

        Beeper (paging) number: _____-_____

    Name of office nurse or assistant: _____

Name of nearest hospital: _____

    Address: _____

    _____

    Hospital phone: _____-_____

    Extension for respiratory-care department: _____

    Name of therapist: _____

Name of equipment supplier: _____

    Name of contact: _____

    Address: _____

    _____

    Phone: (Home) _____-_____ (Work) _____-_____

Name of home-care company: _____

    Name of contact: _____

    Address: _____

    _____

    Phone: (Home) _____-_____ (Work) _____-_____

Name of ambulance service: _____

    Address: _____

    _____

    Phone: _____-_____

Name of church and denomination: _____

    Name of clergy member: _____

    Address: _____

    _____

    Phone: (Home) _____-_____ (Work) _____-_____

Other phone numbers

Fire department

    Address of nearest station: _____

    _____

    Phone: _____-_____

Police department

    Address of nearest precinct: _____

    _____

    Phone: _____-_____

Electricity company phone: _____-_____

Gas company phone: _____-_____

Phone company phone: _____-_____

Other numbers or comments:

_____

_____

C-7, INFORMATION ON YOUR MEDICATIONS

Use additional sheets of paper for more medications.

Name: _____ Date: _____

Brand name of medication: _____

Generic name of medication: _____

Prescribed dose (number of pills): _____

Number of times each day medication should be administered: _____ _____

Action (purpose) for medication: _____

Other instructions or precautions: _____

_____

Name and phone number of pharmacy where medication was purchased:

_____

_____

Brand name of medication: _____

Generic name of medication: _____

Prescribed dose (number of pills): _____

Number of times each day medication should be administered: _____

Action (purpose) for medication: _____

Other instructions or precautions: _____

_____

Name and phone number of pharmacy where medication was purchased:

_____

Brand name of medication: _____

Generic name of medication: _____

Prescribed dose (number of pills): _____

Number of times each day medication should be administered: _____

Action (purpose) for medication: _____

Other instructions or precautions: _____

Name and phone number of pharmacy where medication was purchased:

Energy expenditure in METS

OCCUPATIONAL ACTIVITIES

Activity	METS
Performing receptionist's duties	1.5
Driving a car	1.5
Sitting at a workbench doing light assembly or repair	2.0
Hammering nails	2.0
Driving a large truck	3.0
Bartending	2.5
Working at a gas station	2.7
Scrubbing floors	2.7
Sweeping or raking	2.8
Light welding	3.0
Stocking shelves	3.0
Working on an assembly line	3.5
Rewiring	3.5
Painting or plastering	4.0
Walking a floor (retail sales)	4.0
Bussing dishes	4.2
Working as a car mechanic	4.5
Mowing lawn with a riding mower	2.5
Pushing a power lawn mower	3.2
Pushing a manual lawn mower	6.4
Lifting and carrying objects	
(20 to 40 lb)	4.5
(40 to 60 lb)	6.4
(80 to 100 lb)	8.5
Operating a jackhammer	6.0
Chopping wood	
With a chainsaw	3.0
With a hand axe or saw	6.0
Doing carpentry work	4.0
Doing construction work	5.0
Doing handyman work	5.0
Digging ditches	6.5

LEISURE ACTIVITIES

Activity	METS
Knitting	1.2
Playing cards	1.6
Painting	1.6
Playing the piano	2.1
Playing miniature golf	2.5
Horseback riding at an easy pace	2.5
Power boating	2.5
Playing volleyball	3.5
Fishing	3.0
Bowling	3.0
Wood carving	3.0
Playing horseshoes	3.0
Sailing	3.5
Playing golf, using a power cart	3.5
Playing golf, walking	5.0
Bicycling	4.0
Dancing	4.5
Light gardening	2.0
Performing more difficult tasks of gardening	5.0
Square dancing	4.0
Trout fishing	6.0
Playing tennis	7.0
Roller-skating	7.0
Snow skiing	8.0
Playing handball	12.0
Rowing	12.0

ADL

Activity	METS
Sewing by hand	1.2
Sewing with a machine	1.4
Sweeping floors	1.5
Preparing food while standing	2.0
Ironing while standing	2.5
Dusting	2.5
Vacuuming rugs	2.6
Cleaning windows	2.8
Scrubbing floors	3.0
Washing and drying clothes in a machine	3.4
Changing bed linens	3.4
Straightening rooms (for example, making beds)	2.8
Washing dishes by hand	1.4
Dressing and undressing	2.0
Performing personal-hygiene activities	2.0
Shaving face or combing hair	2.0
Walking	
2 mph	2.0-3.0
3 mph	4.0-5.0
Jogging (10-minute mile)	10.0
Walking up stairs	5.0
Walking down stairs	4.5
Bathing in tub	2.5
Bathing in shower	3.5
Having sexual intercourse	3.5-5.5
Bicycling (9.5 mph)	5.0

Postural-drainage positions for gravity drainage of the airways in the lungs

Positions for segments in the right lung

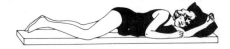

Upper lobe
Posterior segments—left side down, ¾ prone

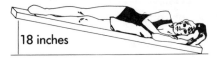

Lower lobe
Lateral-basal segment—left side down, head down ~45°

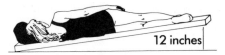

Middle lobe
Medial and lateral segments
Left side down, ¾ supine, head down ~30°

Positions for segments in the left lung

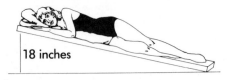

Upper lobe
Posterior segments
Right side down, ¾ prone, head elevated ~45°

Continued.

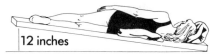

Upper lobe
Lingula—right side down, ¾ supine, head down ~30°

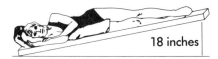

Lower lobe
Lateral-basal—right side down, head down ~45°

Positions for segments in both the right and left lung

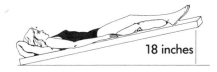

Lower lobes
Anterior medial and basal
Supine, head down ~45°

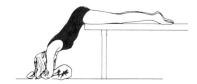

Lower lobes
Posterior basal—prone, head down ~65°

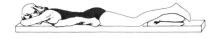

Lower lobes
Superior segments—prone

Continued.

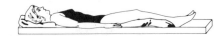

Upper lobes
Anterior segments—supine

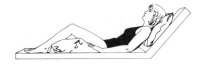

Upper lobes
Apical segment—supine, upright ~65°

AN ALTERNATIVE METHOD OF POSTURAL DRAINAGE

Following are nine postural-drainage positions and the segments and lobes affected by each one.

1. Sitting upright, <65° to supine—drains the apical segment of the upper lobe
2. Supine, flat—drains the anterior segments and upper lobes
3. Supine, head elevated—drains the anterior and apical segments and upper lobes
4. Lying on right side—drains the lateral segment of the left lower lobe and cardiac segment of the right lower lobe
5. Lying on right side, three-fourths prone—drains posterior of the left lower lobe and apical segment
6. Lying on right side, three-fourths supine—drains the lingula and the anterior segment of the left lower lobe
7. Lying on left side—drains the lateral segment of the right lower lobe
8. Lying on left side, three-fourths prone—drains the posterior segment of the right upper lobe and the apical and posterior segments of the right lower lobe
9. Lying on left side, three-fourths supine—drains the right middle lobe and the anterior segment of the right lower lobe

Home medication schedules

Sample medication schedule 1

List each medication and its dosage, as well as all therapies.

Anhydrous theophylline (Theo Dur): 300 mg bid
Metaproterenol sulfate (Alupent): 2 puffs qid
Beclomethasone dipropionate (Vanceril): 2 puffs qid
Digoxin: 0.25 mg qd

Furosemide (Lasix): 5 mg bid
Tetracycline: 0.5 mg qid
O_2 per cannula: 1 L/min

The following chart is for a patient who reports rising at 7 AM and retiring at 10 PM.

Time	Medication	Date:												
7:30 AM	Anhydrous theophylline (1 pill)													
	Metaproterenol sulfate (2 puffs)													
	Beclomethasone dipropionate (2 puffs)													
	Digoxin (1 pill)													
	Furosemide (1 pill)													
	Tetracycline (1 pill)													
	O_2 (1 L/min all day)													
11:30 AM	Metaproterenol sulfate (2 puffs)													
	Beclomethasone dipropionate (2 puffs)													
	Tetracycline (1 pill)													
5 PM	Metaproterenol sulfate (2 puffs)													
	Beclomethasone dipropionate (2 puffs)													
	Tetracycline (1 pill)													
7:30 PM	Anhydrous theophylline (1 pill)													
	Furosemide (1 pill)													
9:30 PM	Metaproterenol sulfate (2 puffs)													
	Beclomethasone dipropionate (2 puffs)													
	Tetracycline (1 pill)													

Comments and reminders:
Wait 1 minute between metaproterenol sulfate puffs and 10 minutes between metaproterenol sulfate and beclomethasone dipropionate puffs.
Wear O_2 continuously at 1 L/min.
Take all prescribed tetracycline pills. Don't save any.
Avoid dairy products when taking a tetracycline pill.
Drink at least 10 glasses of liquid each day. Avoid caffeine and alcohol.

Sample medication schedule 2

Anhydrous theophylline (Theo Dur): 300 mg bid
Metaproterenol sulfate (Alupent): 2 puffs qid
Beclomethasone dipropionate (Vanceril): 2 puffs qid
Digoxin: 0.25 mg qd

Furosemide (Lasix): 5 mg bid
Tetracycline: *
Postural drainage: †

The following chart is for a patient who reports rising at 7 AM and retiring at 10 PM.

Time	Medication	Date:							
7 AM	Anhydrous theophylline (1 tablet)								
	Metaproterenol sulfate (2 puffs)								
	Beclomethasone dipropionate (2 puffs)‡								
	Furosemide (1 tablet)								
	Digoxin (1 tablet)								
11 AM	Metaproterenol sulfate (2 puffs)								
	Beclomethasone dipropionate (2 puffs)‡								
3 PM	Metaproterenol sulfate (2 puffs)								
	Beclomethasone dipropionate (2 puffs)‡								
7 PM	Anhydrous theophylline (1 tablet)								
	Metaproterenol sulfate (2 puffs)								
	Beclomethasone dipropionate (2 puffs)‡								
	Furosemide (1 tablet)								
10 PM	Metaproterenol sulfate (2 puffs)								
	Beclomethasone dipropionate (2 puffs)‡								

Comments and reminders:
*One pill should be administered four times each day when sputum turns green. Drug should not be taken with dairy products. The physician should also be called.
†Drug should be administered twice each day as instructed when amount of sputum increases, when sputum changes color, or when the patient is more short of breath.
‡Drug should be administered 10 minutes after metaproterenol sulfate with 1 minute between all puffs.

List each medication and its dosage, as well as all therapies.

Time	Medication	Date:						

Comments and reminders:

Modified calisthenic exercises

These exercises can be modified to meet the needs of the disabled or deconditioned patient. They are divided into six groups according to the level of energy expenditure. Group I requires the least amount of energy; Group VI requires the highest amount of energy. The first figure in each row shows the starting position, and the next figures show the position to be performed on the first of four counts in the exercise sequence. The rate at which the calisthenics are done can be quickened or slowed to increase or decrease the energy needed to perform an exercise. Generally, 10 to 15 repetitions per minute is an appropriate pace.

Many of these same exercises can be used in ventilation retraining. The focus during VRE would be on breathing control rather than strength or endurance training. If an activity is too difficult, for example, if the patient cannot control ventilation (use the diaphragm and pursed-lip breathing in coordination with the motion of the exercise), it should be modified to allow the patient to concentrate on breathing control during the exercise.

Some figures are included at the end of this appendix (p. 225) to suggest other calisthenics that can be modified and used in training.

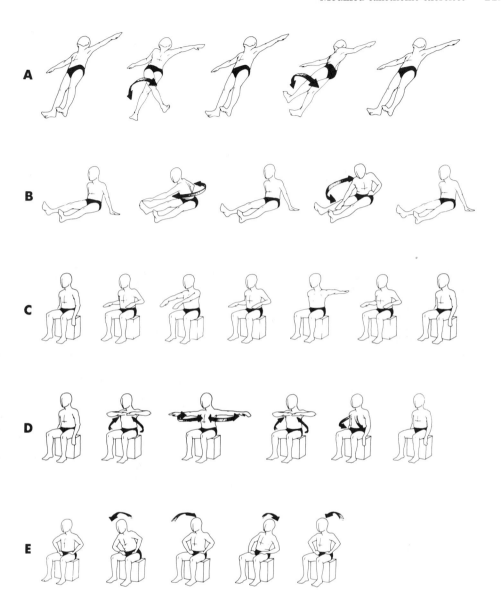

Appendix G-1, Group I.

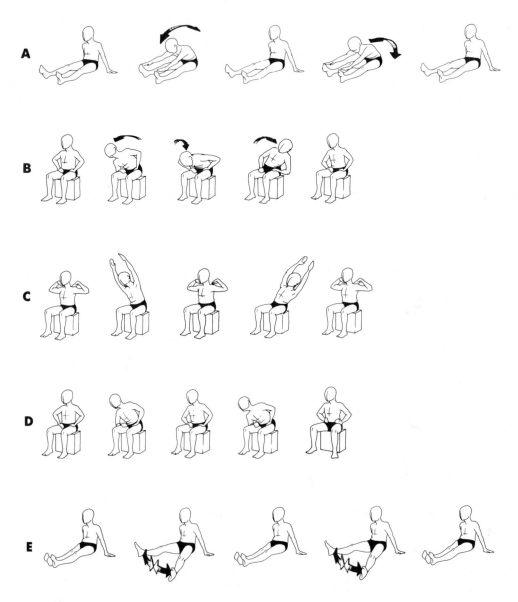

Appendix G-2, Group II.

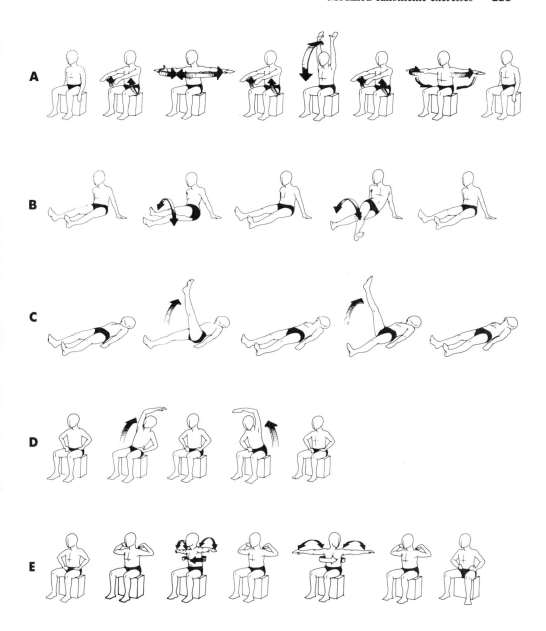

Appendix G-3, Group III.

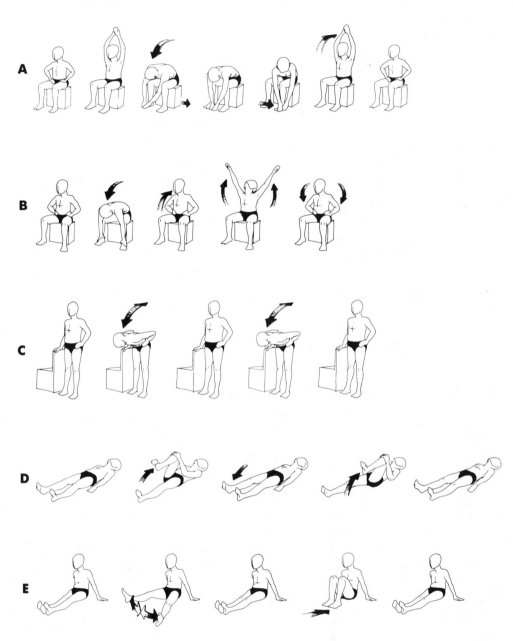

Appendix G-4, Group IV.

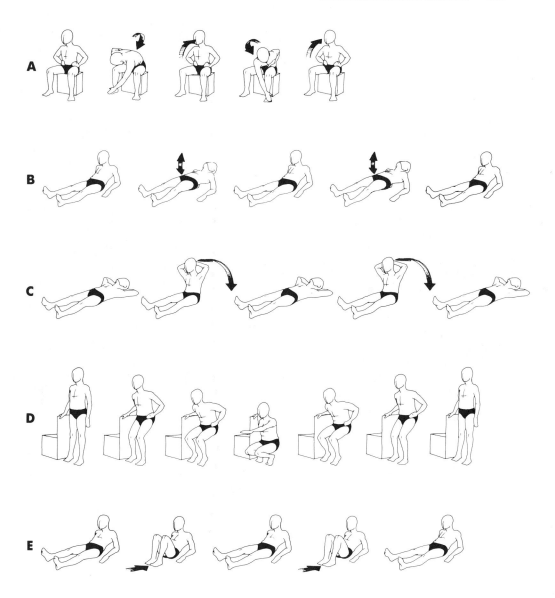

Appendix G-5, Group V.

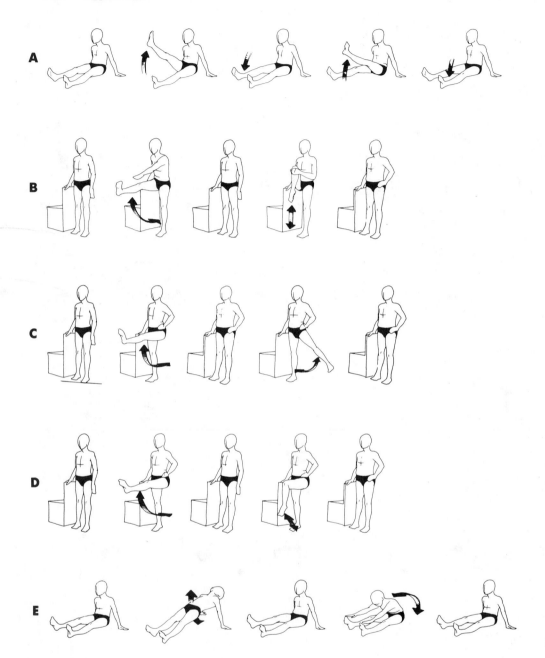

Appendix G-6, Group VI.

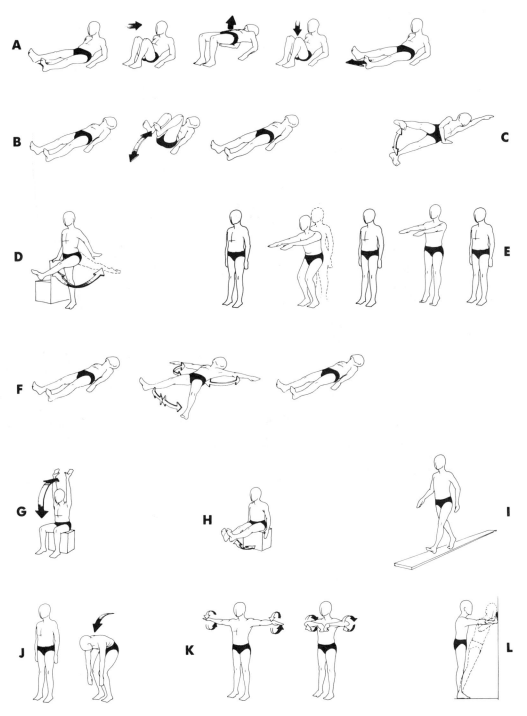

Appendix G-7.

Oxygen cylinders

Table H-1 Approximate duration of compressed-gas cylinders

Cylinder size	Volume of O_2 when full	Flow rate (in hours)				
		1 L/min 60 L/hour	2 L/min 120 L/hour	3 L/min 180 L/hour	4 L/min 240 L/hour	5 L/min 300 L/hour
D	420 qt	6.5*	3.25*	2*	1.5*	1.25*
	396 L	5†	2.5†	1.5†	1.25†	1†
	14 cu/ft	1.5‡	0.75‡	0.5‡	0.33‡	—
E	696 qt	10.25*	5*	3.25*	2.5*	2*
	622 L	7†	4†	2.5†	2†	1.5†
	22 cu/ft	2.25‡	1‡	0.75‡	0.5‡	0.33‡
G	5630 qt	88.75*	44.5*	29.5*	22*	17.75*
	5330 L	69†	34.75†	23†	17.25†	13.75†
	185 cu/ft	19.75‡	9.75‡	6.5‡	>5‡	>4‡
M	3180 qt	57.5*	28.75*	19*	14.25*	11.5*
	3452 L	44.5†	22.25†	14.75†	11†	9†
	122 cu/ft	13‡	6.5‡	4.25‡	3.25‡	<2.5‡
H or K	7320 qt	115.5*	57.75*	38.5*	28.75*	23*
	6930 L	89.25†	44.5†	29.75†	22.25†	17.75†
	244 cu/ft	26‡	13‡	8.75‡	6.5‡	5.25‡

*Duration in hours of full cylinder to completely empty, or 0 psig.
†Duration in hours of full cylinder to 500 psig.
‡Duration in hours of cylinder at 500 psig to 0 psig.
NOTE:
All cylinders are filled to 2200 psig at 70° F.
Air cylinders hold only slightly less than O_2 cylinders, so the difference is ignored.
Aluminum cylinders hold slightly more than alloy cylinders. Refer to calculations in Chapter 7 and Table H-3 to determine duration of aluminum cylinders.

Table H-2 Characteristics of commonly used medical gases and cylinders

Gas	Use	Flammability	U.S. color code	Physical status at 70° F	Cylinder size and capacity			
					4.5 in × 20 in **D**	4.5 in × 30 in **E**	8.5 in × 55 in **G**	9 in × 55 in **H or K**
O_2	Therapy	Supports combustion	Green	~2015 psig* gas	12.5 ft³† (~0.18)	22 ft³† (~0.29)	185 ft³† (~2.4)	244 ft³† (~3.1)
Air ($O_2 + N_2$)	Therapy, industry	Supports combustion	Yellow or black and white	~2015 psig* gas	12.5	22	185	220
CO_2	Therapy, industry	Prevents combustion	Gray	~825 psig liquid or gas	33	56	425	—
Mixture (CO_2-O_2)	Therapy	Supports combustion	Gray and green	~1800 psig gas	12.6	22	185	—
N_2	Laboratory, surgery	Prevents combustion	Black	~1800 psig gas	—	56	—	220
Helium (He)	Pulmonary-function testing, laboratory, industry	Prevents combustion	Brown	~1800 psig gas	10.5	17	150	—
Mixture (He-O_2)	Therapy	Supports combustion	Brown and green	~1800 psig gas	11	18.5	150	—
Nitrous oxide (N_2O)	Anesthesia	Supports combustion	Light blue	~825 psig liquid or gas	34.5	57	485	557
Cyclopropane [$(CH_2)_3$]	Anesthesia	Flammable	Orange or orange and chrome	~75 psig liquid or gas	3.3	30	—	—

*Most cylinders manufactured today are marked with a + on the shoulder. This symbol indicates that the cylinder may be filled to a pressure 10% more than the listed filling pressure (for example, 2015 psig [listed filling pressure] + 201 psig [10% of the listed filling pressure] = 2216 psig [the pressure to which the cylinder can be filled]).

†1 ft³ of gas = 28.3 L.

Table H-3   Tank-use factors*

Factors	D	E	M	G	H or K
L/psig	0.18	0.28	1.57	2.38	3.14
Capacity at 500 psig	90	140	785	1190	1570
Capacity to 500 psig	306	482	2667	4140	5360

*Usage factor $= \dfrac{\text{cu/ft full} \times 28.3 \text{ L/cu/ft}}{\text{psig full}}$

The duration of a cylinder can be calculated at any known pressure from the following equation:

$$\frac{\text{Known tank pressure} \times \text{Tank factor}}{\text{Flow rate}} = \text{Duration (in minutes)}$$

Example: A K cylinder with a pressure of 800 psig operating at 2 L/min

$$\frac{800 \text{ psig} \times 3.14 \text{ L/psig}}{2 \text{ L/min}} = 1256 \text{ min}$$

$$\frac{1256 \text{ min}}{60 \text{ min/hour}} = 20.9 \text{ hours}$$

1981 ATS statement on pulmonary rehabilitation

American Thoracic Society

MEDICAL SECTION OF THE AMERICAN LUNG ASSOCIATION

Pulmonary Rehabilitation

THIS OFFICIAL ATS STATEMENT WAS ADOPTED BY THE ATS EXECUTIVE COMMITTEE, MARCH 1981.

Introduction

The purpose of this statement is to define pulmonary rehabilitation and to describe the essential elements of a pulmonary rehabilitation program. In order to provide comprehensive pulmonary rehabilitation services, a program should be able to carry out the described components of pulmonary rehabilitation and to provide the essential services required as defined in this statement.

Definition of Pulmonary Rehabilitation

Rehabilitation was defined by the Council of Rehabilitation in 1942 as the restoration of the individual to the fullest medical, mental, emotional, social, and vocational potential of which he/she is capable. Instead of addressing solely the physical and mental aspects, rehabilitation should be tailored to maximize one's improvement and minimize the impact of an illness, or a state of progressive deterioration from optimal health, not only on the person, but also his/her family and community.

The American College of Chest Physicians' Committee on Pulmonary Rehabilitation adopted, at its annual meeting in 1974, the following definition:

"Pulmonary rehabilitation may be defined as an art of medical practice wherein an individually tailored, multidisciplinary program is formulated which through accurate diagnosis, therapy, emotional support, and education, stabilizes or reverses both the physio- and psychopathology of pulmonary diseases and attempts to return the patient to the highest possible functional capacity allowed by his pulmonary handicap and overall life situation."

The two principal objectives of pulmonary rehabilitation are to: (*1*) control and alleviate as much as possible the symptoms and pathophysiologic complications of respiratory impairment, and (*2*) teach the patient how to achieve optimal capability for carrying out his/her activities of daily living. Depending on the needs of the specific patient, comprehensive care may include the delivery of a structured, defined "rehabilitation program" as an element of the patient's care. However, in the broadest sense, pulmonary rehabilitation means providing good, comprehensive respiratory care for patients with pulmonary disease. A facility caring for such individuals should be capable of either providing or having access to a regional medical center that is able to offer such a comprehensive care program. The components of pulmonary rehabilitation described in this statement are most useful for patients with chronic obstructive pulmonary disease (COPD), e.g., emphysema, chronic bronchitis, and asthma. However, certain aspects may be selected for patients with other pulmonary disorders.

Sequence of Pulmonary Rehabilitation

A certain sequence should be followed when outlining an appropriate treatment plan. This process involves careful evaluation of the patient, developing a treatment program that best meets the patient's needs, proper assessment of the patient's progress, and a plan for patient follow-up. A logical sequence would proceed as follows:

(*A*) *Patient selection.*
Any patient with symptomatic COPD should be considered for pulmonary rehabilitation. Those patients with either very mild or very severe disease will not generally be placed on as intensive and comprehensive a rehabilitation program as those with moderate to moderately-severe disease.

Multiple factors affect the ultimate success of rehabilitation for any individual. These include, in addition to severity of the disease, the presence of other disabling diseases such as cancer or arthritis, age, intelligence, level of education, occupation, family support, and personal motivation.

(*B*) *Evaluation.*
A careful assessment of the patient should be performed initially. This evaluation would include:
(*1*) *Diagnostic workup.*
Proper identification of the patient's specific respiratory ailment is important because the treatment regimen prescribed should be geared to the patient's disease process. Essential diagnostic information would include: appropriate pulmonary function studies, a chest radiograph, an electrocardiogram, and, when indicated, arterial blood gas measurements at rest and during exercise, sputum analysis and blood theophylline measurements.
(*2*) *Behavioral considerations.*
The best rehabilitation results require personal commitment from the patient, determination and persistence. Additionally, significant psychiatric symptoms of any sort profoundly disrupt compliance. For these reasons, the patient should receive emotional screening assessments and treatment or counseling when required.

Thorough understanding of the disease and its treatment is one of the more important factors in patient motivation, cooperation, and anxiety reduction. This is particularly true in pulmonary rehabilitation during which the patient must master a large amount of knowledge. Yet learning abilities among these patients are often subtly impaired. This can be remedied in two ways: (*a*) Estimating the patient's

Reprinted from AMERICAN REVIEW OF RESPIRATORY DISEASE, Vol. 124, November 1981

Reprinted with permission from The American Lung Association.

learning skills and adjusting the program to the patient's ability, and (b) Requiring the patient to demonstrate new knowledge and skills before progressing further.

The patient must be viewed in terms of the personal and environmental assets at his/her disposal. These include family and social support, potential employment skills, employment opportunities, and community resources. These all need to be evaluated and mobilized for practical help to the patient and to bolster his/her motivation.

(C) *Determine goals.*
It is crucial that short and long-term goals be developed for each individual following the evaluation. The patient and his/her family need to help determine and fully understand these goals, so that they realistically approach the treatment phase.

(D) *Components of pulmonary Rehabilitation.*
(1) *Physical therapy.*
Good bronchial hygiene, e.g., effective coughing, clapping, and bronchial drainage is particularly important to those patients who produce excess mucus within the airways. Pursed-lip breathing may help to slow the respiratory rate and lessen small airway collapse during periods of increased dyspnea. Relaxation techniques can be useful in anxious patients.
(2) *Exercise conditioning.*
A physical conditioning (exercise) program should be considered in any patient with exercise limitations. Selection of appropriate, safe exercise routines is enhanced by measuring workloads, gas exchange behavior, heart rate, and electrocardiogram. However, in selected patients, assessment of the functional work capacity may be possible with such techniques as determining the number of steps the individual can climb or the distance the patient can walk at a certain speed.
(3) *Respiratory therapy.*
Supplemental oxygen and aerosolization of medications such as bronchodilators and corticosteroids are useful for certain patients. In an attempt to limit the inappropriate and excess use of oxygen and respiratory therapy equipment in the home, the American Thoracic Society has developed statements regarding these treatment modalities.

(4) *Education.*
If patient compliance is to be optimized, both the patient and his/her family need to understand the underlying pulmonary disorder. Those individuals outlining the treatment plan should instruct the patient and family about the purpose for medications, as well as their side effects. Proper nutrition, the use and cleaning of respiratory therapy equipment, techniques of physical therapy modalities, and details of an exercise conditioning program must all be carefully explained.
(5) *General.*
The importance of smoking cessation must be emphasized. Attention should be paid to such environmental factors as temperature, humidity, inhaled irritants, and altitude. Although there is little objective data that adequate hydration liquefies airway secretions, it is agreed that dehydration should be prevented. Immunization with the influenza and pneumococcal vaccines is recommended. An appropriate use of such pharmacologic agents as beta$_2$ agonists, methylxanthines, antimicrobials, and corticosteroids is important, and their indications must be understood by the primary care physician.

(E) *Assessment of patient's progress.*
While the treatment plan is being developed, the patient's progress should be monitored. This will help both the patient and the health care team objectively evaluate the plan outlined, so that any needed changes can be initiated.

(F) *Long-term followup.*
Ongoing care will generally be the responsibility of the primary care physician. Periodic reassessment can be beneficial to the patient, as a way of objectively evaluating progress and allowing for educational reinforcement.

Services Required for Pulmonary Rehabilitation

A variety of services are provided through a pulmonary rehabilitation program. Many patients with COPD will not need these services; however, they should be available for those patients with special needs or more severe disease.

(A) *Essential services.*
(1) *Initial medical evaluation and care plan.*

Perform a complete history and physical examination. Obtain appropriate laboratory tests. Make the correct diagnosis. Outline a proper therapy regimen for ongoing care.
(2) *Patient education, evaluation, and program coordination.*
Educate patient regarding lung anatomy and physiology, disease process, useful therapeutic modalities, and other relevant matters. Coordinate allied health personnel involved in the patient's care. Make home visits, as necessary.
(3) *Respiratory therapy techniques.*
Educate patient concerning proper use and cleaning of respiratory therapy equipment. Administer therapy as prescribed by attending physician. Make home visits as needed to insure compliance.
(4) *Physical therapy techniques, including exercise conditioning.*
Educate patient regarding relaxation techniques, proper breathing, clapping, and bronchial drainage. Measure functional work capacity and develop an exercise conditioning program. Record physiologic changes resulting from exercise training.
(5) *Daily performance evaluation.*
Evaluate activities of daily living. Teach energy conservation (work simplification) and self-care techniques.
(6) *Social service evaluation.*
Obtain social history and determine patient's psychosocial assets and needs. Evaluate potential for compliance as well as actual compliance. Mobilize family or other interested individuals as part of extended support system to be used following discharge from the hospital. Evaluate third-party payer problems and help in resolving such problems. Assist in making arrangements for needed community resources, including financial aid, homemaker services, and extended care facilities.
(7) *Nutritional evaluation.*
Evaluate the patient's nutritional status. Outline dietary prescription based on the patient's specific nutritional needs.

(B) *Additional services.*
(1) *Psychological evaluation.*
Administer psychometric battery that includes tests designed to measure organic brain dysfunction, IQ, personality profile, psychosocial assets, impact of illness on person, his/her family, etc. Help patient and family develop coping mechanisms

© AMERICAN LUNG ASSOCIATION, 1981

AMERICAN THORACIC SOCIETY

to control not only chronic anxiety or depression but also acute exacerbations.

(2) Psychiatric evaluation.
Categorize personality pattern. Make psychiatric diagnosis if one exists. Provide specific psychiatric support and/or therapy when needed. If necessary, make specific recommendations regarding optimal psychopharmacologic agents.

(3) Vocational evaluation.
Assess vocational rehabilitation potential for those patients with significant impairment. Includes vocational tests, interviews, on-the-job observation, as well as determining whether the subject has the work capacity to meet the oxygen requirements of his/her job. Work output can generally be sustained for an eight-hour period if one does not exceed 30-40% of his/her attained maximum oxygen consumption.

A physician knowledgeable about respiratory diseases should perform the initial complete examination and assist in outlining a proper regimen of treatment.

The specific provider for the other services may vary from program to program. A multidisciplinary team that might include a professional nurse, respiratory therapist, physical therapist, occupational therapist, dietitian, social worker, and pulmonary or cardiopulmonary technologist expert in pulmonary rehabilitation techniques is appropriate for those settings where large numbers of patients are referred and for teaching or research purposes. However, in other settings, it may be possible to provide similar services with fewer individuals if they are highly-qualified and specially-trained in evaluation and management of the patient with COPD. In selected patients, the evaluation and delivery of a comprehensive care program can be accomplished in an outpatient setting. Thus, the techniques of rehabilitation should be within the reach of all physicians, applying the principles expressed in this document.

Benefits and Limitations of Pulmonary Rehabilitation

(A) Benefits.
A comprehensive respiratory care program can result in definite benefits to the patient. There is overwhelming evidence that a comprehensive respiratory care program can result in an improved quality of life and a significantly improved capability for carrying out his/her daily activities.

Participation in a comprehensive pulmonary rehabilitation program has repeatedly been shown to decrease the hospital days required per patient per year. Some patients may be able to return to useful employment, thus making a contribution to the work force. Patients can achieve a significant reduction in anxiety, depression, and somatic concern with an associated improvement in their own ego strength. Numerous studies have shown that the physical conditioning of patients with COPD can be substantially improved with a regular exercise training program.

Cessation of smoking can result in improved pulmonary function, reduction of cough, decreased sputum production, and lessened dyspnea. The course of COPD may be altered if the airway abnormality is detected early.

(B) Limitations.
Event though all of the above benefits have been documented, an extension of lifespan and slowing of pulmonary function deterioration have not been shown in the majority of published studies. Through the use of routine office spirometry, COPD can be detected at a much earlier stage when institution of a comprehensive respiratory care program may more effectively achieve an alteration in the patient's course.

A significant problem relates to the fact that only approximately 20-35% of the participants in smoking cessation programs quit permanently. More effort needs to be applied to the prevention of respiratory disease, rather than concentrating on treatment after significant disability has occurred.

Another major factor interfering with delivery of good care is the unevenness in our capacity to deliver community-based services. A visiting nurse association (or its equivalent) does not exist in every community, nor do socially-oriented service programs, such as Meals on Wheels, Homemaker's, etc.

Which tests are required to appropriately determine impairment/disability needs to be more clearly determined. Ideally, patients should be adequately evaluated and treated comprehensively *prior to* a final disability determination.

Conclusion

In the 17th century, Jeremy Taylor said, "To preserve a man alive in the midst of so many diseases and hostilities, is as great a miracle as to create him." In the past, rehabilitation has been applied rather loosely to vaguely describe various approaches to long-term management of the chronically ill patient. The time has come for us to not only define what we mean by pulmonary rehabilitation but to describe the essential services required. This comprehensive approach to patient evaluation will result in improved care for respiratory patients so that they may be restored to their most optimal potential.

This statement was prepared by an *ad hoc* committee of the Scientific Assembly on Clinical Problems. The committee members are as follows:

JOHN E. HODGKIN, *Chairman*
MICHAEL J. FARRELL
SUZANNE R. GIBSON
RICHARD E. KANNER
IRVING KASS
LAWRENCE M. LAMPTON
MARGARET NIELD
THOMAS L. PETTY

References

1. Masferrer R, O'Donohue WJ Jr., Seriff NS, *et al.* Home use of equipment for patients with respiratory disease [ATS Statement]. Am Rev Respir Dis 1977; 115:893-5.

2. Block AJ, Burrows B, Kanner RE, *et al.* Oxygen administration in the home [ATS Statement]. Am Rev Respir Dis 1977; 115:897-9.

3. California Thoracic Society guidelines for pulmonary rehabilitation, a statement by the CTS Respiratory Care Assembly. Newsletter, Respiratory Care Assembly of California Thoracic Society, September 1979, 8(#1).

4. Daughton DM, Fix AJ, Kass I, *et al.* Physiological-intellectual components of rehabilitation success in patients with chronic obstructive pulmonary disease (COPD). J Chronic Dis 1979; 32:405-9.

5. Hodgkin JE, ed. Chronic Obstructive Pulmonary Disease. Current Concepts in Diagnosis and Comprehensive Care. Park Ridge, Ill: American College of Chest Physicians, 1979.

6. Hodgkin JE. Pulmonary rehabilitation. In: Simmons D, ed, Current Pulmonology III. New York: John Wiley & Sons, 1981.

7. Intermittent positive pressure breathing (IPPB). Clin Notes Respir Dis, Winter 1979, pp. 3-6.

8. Kimbel P, Kaplan AS, Alkalay I, *et al.* An in-hospital program for rehabilitation of patients with chronic obstructive pulmonary disease. Chest 1971; 60(Suppl):6s-10s.

9. Lertzman MM, Cherniack RM. Rehabilitation of patients with chronic obstructive pulmonary disease. Am Rev Respir Dis 1976; 114: 1145-65.

10. Moser KM, Bokinsky GE, Savage RT, Archibald CJ, Hansen PR. Physiological and functional effects of a comprehensive rehabilitation program upon patients with chronic obstructive pulmonary disease. Arch Int Med 1980; 140:1596-1601.

AMERICAN THORACIC SOCIETY

11. Nield M. The effect of health teaching on the anxiety level of patients with chronic obstructive lung disease. Nursing Res 1971; 20:537-41.

12. Petty TL, ed. Chronic Obstructive Pulmonary Disease. New York: Marcel Dekker, Inc., 1978.

13. Petty TL. Pulmonary rehabilitation, Basics of RD. New York: American Thoracic Society, 1975.

14. Pierce AK, Paez PN, Miller WF. Exercise therapy with the aid of a portable oxygen supply in patients with emphysema. Am Rev Respir Dis 1965; 91:653-9.

15. Skills of the Health Team Involved in Out-of-Hospital Care for Patients with COPD, a statement by the Section on Nursing, Scientific Assembly on Clinical Problems, American Thoracic Society. ATS News 1977; 3:18.

Index _____

Page numbers in *italics* indicate illustrations and boxed material. Page numbers followed by a *t* indicate tables.